AUTISM IS A BLESSING

Charlie

Robyn-
Thank you for all your help c̄ our students.
You are a blessing.

AUTISM IS A BLESSING

A Family's Struggle with Autism and How They Found the Blessings

Patty Corrigan Myers

TATE PUBLISHING & *Enterprises*

AUTISM IS A BLESSING

A Family's Struggle with Autism and How They Found the Blessings

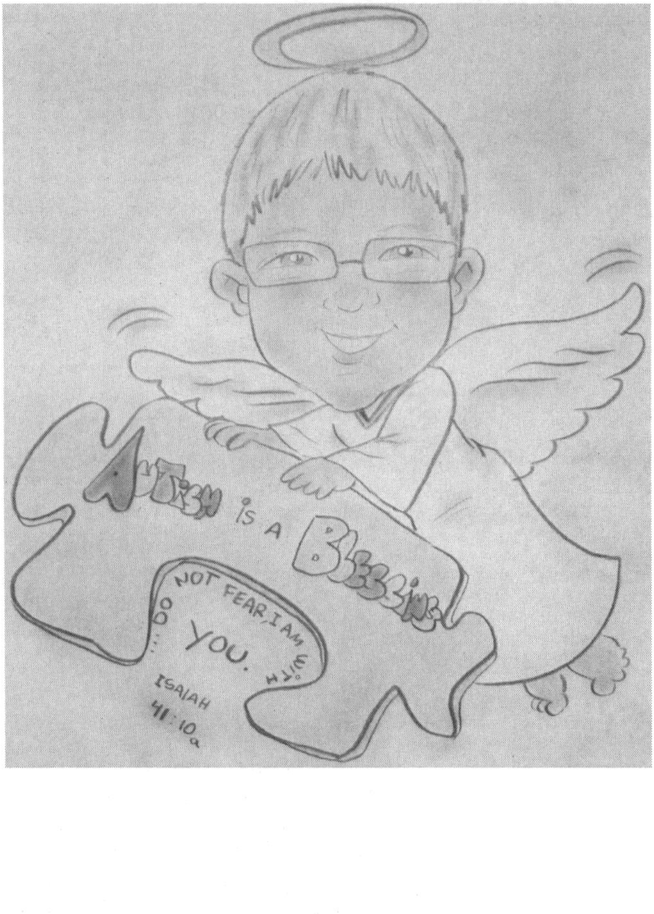

This title is also available as a Tate Out Loud product. Visit www.tatepublishing.com for more information.

Published by Tate Publishing & Enterprises, LLC
127 E. Trade Center Terrace | Mustang, Oklahoma 73064 USA
1.888.361.9473 | www.tatepublishing.com

Tate Publishing is committed to excellence in the publishing industry. The company reflects the philosophy established by the founders, based on Psalm 68:11,
"The Lord gave the word and great was the company of those who published it."

Cover & Interior Design Jonathan Lindsey

Published in the United States of America

ISBN: 978-1-60696-264-0
1. Medical: autism 2. memoir: reference
08.09.17

DEDICATION

I would like to dedicate this book to my son, Charlie. You are my inspiration, you are my hope. You have taught me so much in your six short years so far...keep teaching me. I pray that God continues to use you for *his* glory. I love you son.

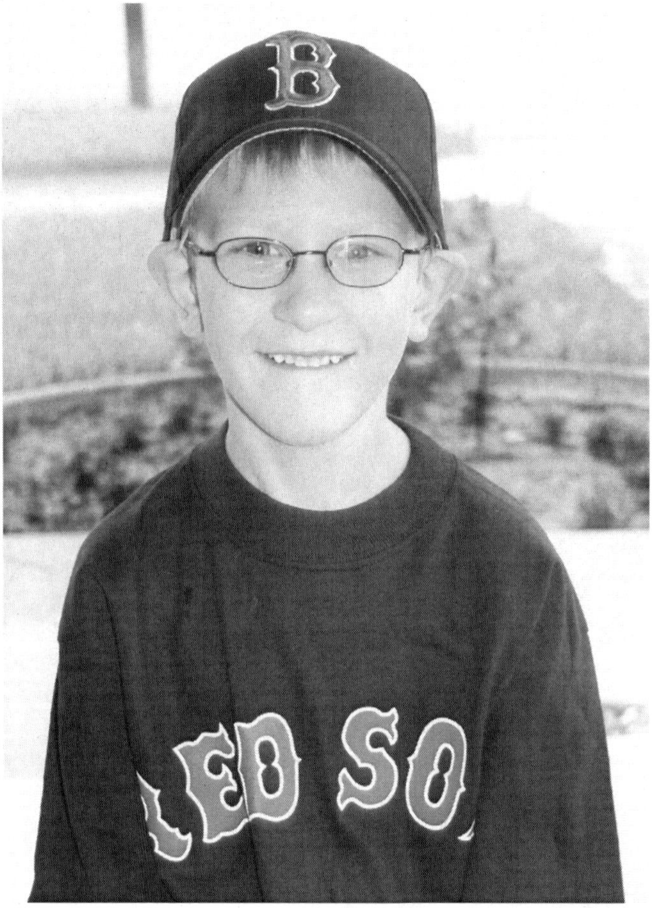

Charles Nicholas Myers

ACKNOWLEDGEMENTS

To Claudia, one of my good friends who has really been there for me. We became friends when we worked together in the fall of 1993, right after my father passed away. No matter what struggle I was going through or how much I didn't keep in touch because I was sad, scared, confused, and wanted to be alone, she never stopped being there for me. She never took it personally, if I didn't call for a while, she was just *always* there. I would ramble emails to her and tell her what a tough day I had with Charlie, and she would be so supportive. I thank her so much for that, because in the end, all we need is someone we know, no matter what, in the good and the bad, is always going to be there for us. Thank you, Claudia.

Carlie (Mrs. Fucci) was another person that has really helped me through this journey with Charlie. I have known her since I was 13 or 14. She and her husband, Tom, have always been there for me and have been great, Godly examples to look up to. I called her about a month or so after we learned of Charlie's diagnosis to have her help out in our office. I already had Gigi helping me for over three years, but knowing this about Charlie and having to take him to several therapy appointments and doctor's visits, I needed some more help and support. I also didn't want to put too much on Gigi because she was my rock at our company. Carlie came to help out, and I was also wanting to help her out as well. She had lost her husband Tom, December 22, 2001. We both needed to help each other. She has sat many a time and listened to me sob and grieve, and has just been there without judging me. I thank her so much for coming to help me at one of the lowest times in my life, and for just being there for me to talk to and get out my feelings. Besides my husband's cancer and my father's death, hearing that my son had autism was one of the worst days of my life. I always felt loved when I was with her, and she seemed to always have the most comforting words when times were tough. She gives the best hugs and has encouraged me in my walk with the Lord. Thank you, Carlie.

Dodie is an old friend from high school that has lived in the Orlando area for more than 10 years, and we were able to connect again when we moved here too. She has been a steady companion and friend through such a difficult time. She will call me even if I don't want to talk and will leave a prayer for me on my answering machine. She has been a great, Christian friend and example of God's grace through trials. She has had many trials of her own to overcome and knows God's grace personally. Dodie has stood by me when I wasn't feeling so good but still encouraged me to press on. Thank you, Dodie.

Ms. Sirlon, you were only able to help and teach Charlie a few months, but you were such a crucial part of his progress and our support in those first few difficult months. Thank you for your knowledge, your big smile that would greet us everyday at school, your advice, and most of all, your listening ear. We hated to leave you; it broke our hearts. Tony and I will never forget what you did to help Charlie, and we will always remain close to you. Thank you, Ms. Sirlon.

Ms. Jessica, you were Charlie's first speech therapist. We came to you only a few weeks after being told our son had autism. We were scared about the future. I would always ask you: what will he will be like, would other kids like him, and how were other kids doing as they've grown? You would always remind me that you didn't know, but I should be positive and stay focused on the goal of getting him to communicate. You were with me when he said his first words after so many years. You sat with me as we both had tears coming down our cheeks when he finally signed and said "more" at the age of three. Thank you so much for teaching me patience and to not look too far ahead and to just focus on today. Even when he screamed almost the entire time in therapy, you helped me to see that we can get through anything with time and patience. You will always be a part of Charlie's family pictures, and I will always show him your picture and tell him how much you did for him and his parents. Thank you, Jessica.

Our former home, Bible-Study group, has been great. We joined our pastor's group in August of 2005 and loved it. I have learned so much about God's word and love for me in that time. The support I have gotten from the people in that group has been tremendous. I have also learned the most from Gina and Chuck. Our pastor and his wife have a son who has autism. He is 15 now, and they have been such a positive and powerful example to Tony and me. We see their patience, love, steadfastness, control, hopefulness, and their encouragement with their son. We follow their lead. Thank you for listening to me cry and helping me to figure out that God is always with us and right beside us. As Gina would say to me so often, "this too shall pass." Thank you Michael, Mary, Tory, Adam, Grant, Julie, Sean, Andrea, Lori, Lynn, Lee, Violet, Juan, Roger, Chuck, and Gina.

To my friend Kristina, you have been there with me since we were in the seventh grade. We have had a lot of struggles that have seemed to fall around the same time, and it has been difficult to be there for each other at certain times. I want to thank you for your love and support. Just know that God is always holding *your* hand and carrying *you* through *your* difficult trials as well. You also have been blessed. Thank you, Kristina.

To my neighbor, Gigi, you will probably never know how much you helped my son and me. Thank you for helping me and always giving love to my son. I really feel strongly that you helped him to come out of his "shell" every time you were around Charlie. Your love and hugs helped him in those early days more than you will ever know. Finally at four years old he could answer the question; "how old are you?" after asking him almost every day since he was born. It took four years, but he can do it. Also, thank you for helping with our business. I could have never made it without you. Thank you, Gigi.

To Troy, thank you for all of the confidence you gave me when I first approached you about writing a book. I remember you told me that everyone is a writer. Thank you for taking the time to encourage me and give me advice along the way. It really meant so much to me.

To Gary and Lawrence, these are the two guys that bought our home-therapy company in November, 2004. I want to thank you both so much for taking it over, which allowed me to help my children and especially Charlie. I could not have kept doing what I was doing. You guys probably saved me in so many ways, mentally and physically. Thank you for your patience at such a difficult time in our lives. You will always be a part of our family because you were an integral part in our transition to give Charlie a better chance in life. Thank you, Gary and Lawrence.

To Danny, our friend and attorney. What can we say? You kept us strong and calm as needed. You prayed with us. Thanks for your support and love. Thank you, Danny.

To my brother and sisters, you have been a great support. We have always stuck together even when the times were tough. Only we know what struggles we each have overcome, and God will use *each* one to help others. Thank you for your listening ears and shoulders to rely on for comfort. Thank you, Kelly, John, and Jenny.

To my half brothers,...since our dad died, I have slowly gotten to know you all even more. I am so glad I finally got to meet Jeff. We will always be connected to each other. Thanks Jeff, Barry, Don, and Dan.

To my mom, thank you for trying to understand what autism is and for being supportive in those tough times of stress and worry. Thank you for always trying to help out when you could. You are the only grandma that Charlie has. Thank you, Mom.

To Ms. Kim, Ms. Trish, Ms. Lisa, Ms. Kaak and Ms. Sherry, I can't thank you all enough for being such a great team to help my son in his kindergarten class (the first time around). He blossomed so much in that year. You all will *always* be a part of our scrapbook. Thanks for your patience with my son and especially me. Thanks for helping me to be consistent with the potty training...we are still going strong. Thank you, Ms. Kim, Ms. Lisa, Ms. Sherry, Ms. Kaak and Ms. Trish.

To Tory, thank you so much for helping me with the editing. You always were such an inspiration when I would update you on how the writing was going. Thanks so much for the time you took to help me get this out. It has meant a whole lot to me. You can do it girl. It is your turn now. Thank you, Tory.

To my "Pod Girls," you all have gotten me through some tough times. I couldn't make it without your support and love. Thank you, Sharon, Sylvia, Natalie, Lena, Samantha, Donna, Brenda and Jen.

To my daughter Chelsea, I know you have had a tough time watching Charlie struggle. You have helped him so much. Sorry you had to miss out on some things because we would have to leave due to Charlie having a tantrum and being on sensory overload. Thank you for your patience and help with him when you could tell I was at the end of my rope. You will always be his biggest supporter in life. Just keep on loving him as you have done, and he will be ok. Thank you, Chelsea.

My husband Tony, what can I say? We have had eighteen years of marriage and are still going strong. You have been my rock. You have had to put up with a whole lot. Thank you for your love and patience with me especially when I am struggling. With God's help we created two beautiful children. Thank you for your constant love and showing me how to love even more. You have taught me so much in life. I am still learning, so don't stop teaching. You caught my eye the first time we met with your humor, and still make me laugh even in the tough times. Thank you for your leadership and especially your shoulder. Thank you for always being positive even when it looked so stormy. I feel really strongly that one day I will be looking out at you and Charlie playing football together or you and Charlie fishing from the boat. You have gone through a whole lot since we have been married. You lost both parents, uncles, had two surgeries for cancer, and found out your son has autism. Yet you still keep smiling and showing us hope. As we like to tell Charlie constantly; *You can do it. You are a winner*! I will love you forever and ever. Thank you, Tony.

TABLE OF CONTENTS

INTRODUCTION

This is the story of my family's journey with autism. Autism is a brain disorder that was first identified as a specific disorder in 1943 by child psychiatrist Dr. Leo Kanner. It affects a person's ability to communicate, to reason, and to interact with others. It is a spectrum disorder that affects each individual differently and to varying degrees of severity. It is often found in combination with other disabilities. There are three "autism spectrum disorders." They are: Autistic disorder, Aspergers Disorder, and Pervasive Developmental Disorder-Not Otherwise Specified, (PDD-NOS). There is no specific medical test or procedure that can confirm if a person has autism. While some tests can be run to rule out a physical problem, autism is diagnosed by observation. Autism is becoming epidemic. According to the National Institute of Health and the Autism Society of America, autism is the most widely diagnosed developmental disability in the nation, affecting one in 150 children and one in every 94 boys according to the Centers for Disease Control and Prevention. Autism is more common than childhood cancer, cystic fibrosis, and multiple sclerosis combined. It is a lifelong disability. Today alone, 50 families in America will find out that their child has autism. Also, there has been evidence that there are three to four boys being diagnosed for every girl that is diagnosed with autism. The number of children diagnosed with autism has jumped 10 times higher in the last 20 years. There are about 130,000 kids with autism from ages six to 17 in public schools around the country.

It is found equally in all walks of life and in all populations and races around the world. Autism does not discriminate. Its numbers have risen consistently across the United States. Autism spectrum disorders occur in all racial, ethnic, and socioeconomic groups. The thinking and learning abilities of people with autism spectrum disorders can vary—- from gifted to severely challenged. An autism spectrum disorder typically begins before the age of three and lasts throughout a person's life. Research has shown that early intervention can greatly improve a child's development.

The Autism Society of America distributes a pamphlet. The front cover explains the whole story of how autism feels to those affected. It reads as follows:

> Imagine ... If you were unable to communicate
>
> Imagine ... If you were in pain but couldn't tell anyone
>
> Imagine ... If you felt distracted, frustrated, obsessed, and frightened, but You didn't know why
>
> Imagine ... Feeling this way all day, every day

Imagine …Trying to live with an Autism Spectrum Disorder

My objective with this book is to take you through our family's journey and to show you that God is holding your hand the whole time. Some days it may not feel that way, but I can assure you that he is. You *can* get through this! I want to give you some resources and support as you or a loved one travels this journey as well. One of the hardest things that our family had to endure was just understanding what autism was and how it was going to impact our lives. I remember leaving that doctor's office after he diagnosed Charlie's autism and not knowing where to turn or what to do. In this book, I want to give you the information so that you can know where to turn and what to do. Some of my thoughts may be similar to yours and may help you to feel some comfort. Don't feel that you are the only person on this planet with these struggles.

I have always told my husband that I think we, as parents of a child with autism, are in our own special club. Only we understand (in different ways) what it is like to live with autism. Only we understand what it is like to watch your child scream for hours on end curled up in a ball in the corner somewhere and have no idea what is wrong and realize that nothing will stop him from screaming. Only we understand how exciting it was, when at four years old, our child said, "help!" Only we understand how it breaks our heart to see him scream in fear as he hears the electric razor getting ready to role over his head. Only we understand how blessed we are to have Charlie and what he has taught us so far in this journey. Throughout this book, I will also share thoughts of others who live with autism. They will share how autism has been a blessing in their lives and the different experiences they have had with autism.

SOMETHING WAS JUST NOT RIGHT

For this boy I prayed
I Samuel 1:27 (NIV)

When my son Kaelob was 18 months old he went through this complete change. A once happy and content baby suddenly cried constantly. His smile was replaced by tears and then came the violence. He would scream, bang his head off of floors and walls, scratch me and my parents until blood was drawn. He bit, he fought, but what shocked us the most was that he stopped talking. I no longer heard "Mommy" come from his lips.

Jessica (mom)

The pain was excruciating. I had been up all night with awful cramping. I had tossed and turned since five that evening. I took a bath to try and relieve the pain, but even that didn't help. Finally, at three in the morning, I woke up my husband Tony and said, "We need to go to the hospital. I can't stand the pain." The previous day had been my due date, so I knew it was time. Tony took our daughter to our neighbor Gigi's house while I tried to get ready to leave. I was terrified, even though I had had a baby exactly six years and one day ago. I had been nauseas all night and was exhausted because I hadn't slept. We got my bag together and got in the car quickly. My husband seemed a little anxious seeing me in such discomfort. I was saying lots of prayers for the pain and pressure to go away.

Tony drove right through the first red light we came to. Needless to say, I became a little irritated because, unlike me, I needed him to be calm and controlled. We arrived at the hospital. The admitting staff began asking me all these questions. My husband told me I was rude but I felt so nauseas, and I could hardly concentrate on the questions and could not think of the answers. Even though I had done this once before, I will still anxious and scared. They wheeled me upstairs where the nurse there continued with her line of questioning. I thought it would never end. They put all kinds of monitors on me to check the baby and me. I was only dilated about one centimeter. I wanted to cry. I wanted this to be over. The nurse told me to walk around and see if that made my labor progress. We walked around the entire hospital while I sucked on a peppermint to try and relax. I remember being tired of watching the same television news pieces over and over again. Finally they gave me my own room and started administering Pitocin to start my labor.

> I learned that when I set out to teach Vincent how to survive in this world, he gave me a new perspective on how it looked to him. The things that I had taken for granted suddenly became

> new again. Books that "talked" were not the norm. Technology and the cutting-edge society we live in made them a household word. The world was full of sights and sounds that became part of our everyday "chaos" that seemed to take a background seat to the "urgency" of the moment.
>
> Mrs. G. (mother)

We had decided to be surprised about what we were having this time. We already had a beautiful, auburn-haired, blue-eyed little girl. This would probably be our last child no matter the sex. It was fun not knowing, although people would come up to me constantly telling me I "looked" like I was going to have a boy. I also felt strongly that I was having a boy. The television was on in the room to keep my attention off of the labor pains. They started the Pitocin around eleven that morning. The only reason I remember the time was because *The Price is Right* had just started. The first hour, I thought, no problem I can deal with this slight discomfort. Then around 12:30 the pain started coming closer and more intensely. I would hold onto the side of the bed to help it subside. Finally, around 2:00, I told my husband that I couldn't endure the pain and started crying. I said, "I need those drugs!" He called the nurse. She paged the "epidural man," but he took 30 minutes to arrive. Those 45 minutes were the longest of my life. I kept reminding myself that my sister-in-law, Lori had done this without pain medicine and I could do this. Then I said, "She was crazy!" The nurse helped me breath through the contractions. Rationally, I knew that women do this all the time without drugs but there was no way I was going to be able to do it. I would grab a washcloth Tony got me and would squeeze it as tight as possible. As soon as one subsided, another came. I couldn't get relief.

Finally the "epidural man" arrived. He was telling jokes and asking more questions. He was taking his own sweet time. I was so irritated by him, but had to keep my cool or I wouldn't get the pain medication. I couldn't answer his questions I was in so much pain. I gave my husband a dirty look like, "You better answer these questions for me or I will pull all the hair off your chest!" He gave me the anesthesia, and I asked for more because I was still so uncomfortable. The doctor refused and informed me that I needed to feel to be able to push. I wanted to knock him out. He had no idea what it felt like then. Needless to say, I was not too thrilled with him at this point. I tried my best to concentrate on a picture of a beautiful beach or something soothing to relieve the horrible pressure.

They let me rest for an hour or so and then my Obstetrician, Dr. McEachrane came in. He was in full scrubs, mask, and gear. When I saw him looking like that I knew it would only be minutes. All of a sudden, I felt a burst of energy. I was so ready now. I pushed for only three or four times, and there *he* was. My husband screamed, "It's a boy!" I was so happy because I knew he really wanted a boy. I thought, *thank you God, I don't have to do this ever again.*

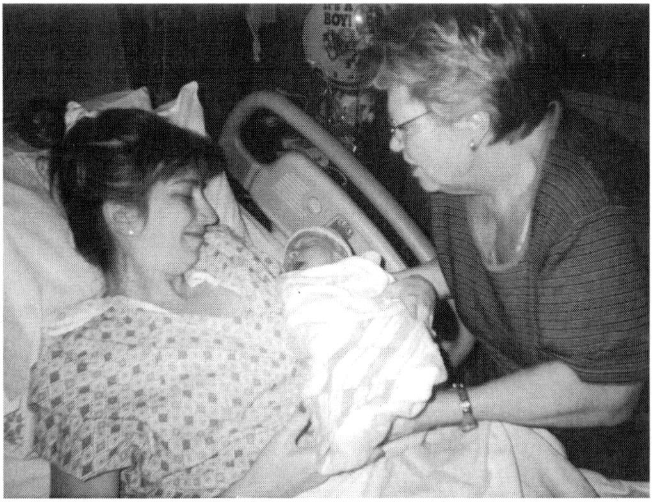

Carlie Fucci and me with Charlie just minutes after he was born July 11, 2001

Our baby was so beautiful. He was perfectly healthy, ten fingers and ten toes. He had cute dimples and big, blue eyes. I was surprised he didn't have red hair like our daughter Chelsea. I cried like a baby just as I had done when my daughter was born. What a miracle it was to witness this. The nurses brought me downstairs to my own room, and I was wiped out. I hadn't slept in more than 24 hours.

Mr. and Mrs. Fucci, our very close, family friends, were right beside me. Mr. Fucci wasn't up to going, but was coaxed by his wife. He was battling kidney disease and walking on a cane. I think he had dialysis that day and was really tired, but Mrs. Fucci insisted that they go to the hospital. They were the first to see Charlie. About thirty minutes after his birth. I loved that they were there, and then soon after, their daughter Kristina came too.

> My husband and I have learned so much about Autism, and we have learned no two kids are alike. We are involved in our son's life 120 percent, from making sure that his needs are met at home and at school. Being able to live an independent life someday, when we are no longer here, is my wish for my child. We believe it is very important for us as parents to help our children reach their full potential, and to educate our communities that these children are also children of God.
>
> Matha (mother)

Our neighbor Gigi brought our daughter in the room. She looked so grown up. I had just seen her about 14 hours ago but somehow she looked like she had grown so much in that short time. She had a beautiful, flowered, white dress and a matching headband. Her beautiful, long, red hair was perfectly curled. Chelsea had the biggest smile on her face when she saw her brother for the first time. She wouldn't say much. She just kept staring at him and smiling with the biggest grin on her face. We had settled on two boy names and decided to let Chelsea pick between them. When she came in the room I asked her to look at him and tell us what his name should be. She said, "Charlie." We all smiled with tears in our eyes.

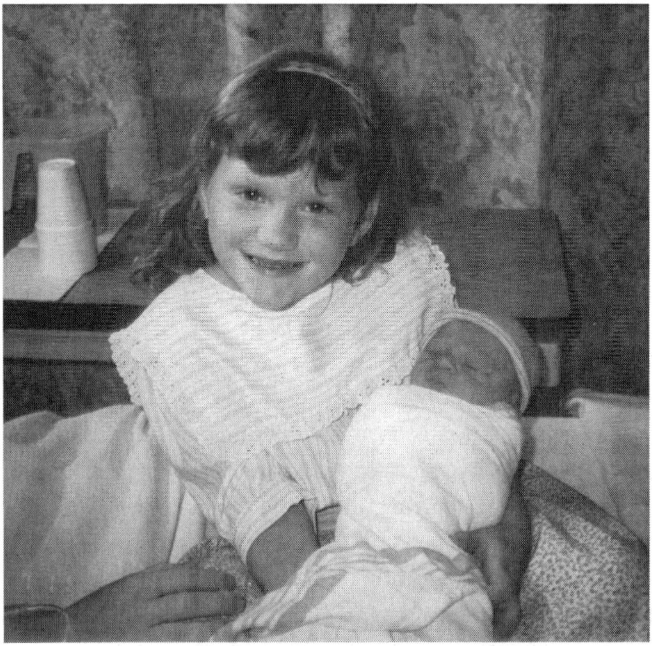

Chelsea meets her brother for the first time.

The next morning, the nurses said Charlie looked a little jaundiced. I thought so too. They let us take him home when I was discharged though. Tony and I would keep an eye on him. We had to take him to the doctor every day for five days to make sure the jaundice was decreasing. Dr. Martell said, if by the fifth day he was still jaundiced, he would have to hospitalize him. Tony and I were nervous the next morning, but sure enough, the jaundice had dropped one point, so he was home free.

The next few weeks were uneventful. I breast fed him for almost four weeks but then had to stop. I felt he needed more than I could give. He would nurse for over 45 minutes and still wanted to eat more. Needless to say I was worn out and sore. I cried to Tony that I couldn't do it anymore so we started giving him formula. He did well with it immediately. I on the other hand, was miserable for at least a week. I still had milk coming in two weeks later.

As soon as all seemed well with Charlie, a month later he started to have a fever and diarrhea. We called the doctor right away and he said to just watch him for the next day and alert him if it got worse. Tony slept beside Charlie all night in the bassinet to watch his fever. Charlie woke up almost every hour and Tony gave him Tylenol every four hours to try and cool the fever.

We went to the airport in the morning and picked up my mom who was arriving from Arizona to see her grandson for the first time. When we got home, Tony changed Charlie's diaper and there was blood. We were terrified. Tony called Dr. Martell and he said that Charlie should be seen immediately. Tony had to go to work and see his patients (he is a physical therapist assistant) since he had spent the morning traveling to and from the airport. My mom and I took Charlie to the doctor. As soon as Dr. Martell saw Charlie, he took his temperature. It was 101. For a four-week-old infant that is a red flag. He said very calmly that Charlie must be taken to the emergency room immediately. He was afraid of sepsis, which is an infection in your bloodstream, or maybe even some brain damage if the fever got too high. All I heard was *brain damage* over and over again.

> There are many challenges that we will always face. We sometimes get discouraged because we never have time alone, we have to scope out restaurants before we can ever go out in case there is something that might upset her, we

> don't have a lot of people qualified to babysit, and it's heartbreaking when she turns violent against the people that love her the most, with no regard to their feelings. We know it's not her fault, but it still hurts.
>
> Jennifer (mother)

I asked Charlie's doctor if we could take him home that same night, and he said he would have to stay for a few days and have some tests run to determine what was wrong. I went blank. I was in shock. My baby could have brain damage? The doctor then looked at me and asked if I was okay? Maybe I looked pale or something, or maybe he could tell I was freaking out. I didn't know what to think. My mind was racing. It felt like an out of body experience. I could hear everyone talking and telling me my instructions, but I was in a fog.

My mom and I went directly across the street to the emergency room. They took him back to the nurse's area and took some blood, x-rays, and then performed a spinal tap. They put an IV line in his arm, which took several nurses to do because he was screaming and fighting so much. It really broke my heart to see my baby going through this. The spinal tap was the toughest to watch because they had to hold him down with force while he screamed very loudly. They insert a needle in his back. I was okay until I saw that, which made me cry. It hit me, at that moment that he was in trouble. I didn't want to call Tony until I knew what was going on. On my mom's insistence, finally I called Tony to tell him. He was in shock and at first thought I was actually joking. I think we both expected to get some medicine from the doctor and be done. Tony arrived later that afternoon. I was exhausted at this point. I don't even think my mom or I had eaten anything yet. They took us up to a regular room an hour or so later. Meanwhile Mom had to be exhausted. She had flown from Arizona to Florida and gone straight to the doctor's office with me and been with me ever since.

The doctor finally arrived around 8 p.m. or so, to tell us she had reviewed the blood work. Charlie had salmonella poisoning. *What*? How could he have salmonella poisoning? We were always careful handling him. I had always heard you could get salmonella poisoning from raw eggs and raw chicken. We tried to think of anything he could have swallowed. Then we remembered that our neighbor's daughter Jasmin had recently gotten a baby chick from her grandfather. My daughter Chelsea had played with it. Could she have touched Charlie after she touched the chick? Charlie stayed in the hospital four days. Tony and I would take shifts. He would stay all night and I would stay during the day. Charlie was on antibiotics all that time which concerned me. Dr. Martell told Tony that we were really lucky that this had not turned out to be a lot worse. He was very, very sick.

> My husband and I are the grandparents of a beautiful non-verbal, autistic child, Sydney. After living in Illinois all of our lives, we chose to move to Fort Wayne in order to help our daughter and husband with their precious little girl who lives one hour east of us. In less than one year, doors have opened including ABA schooling for four-year old Sydney. After seven weeks at the center, Sydney's behavior is improving and she is learning to sign. This has not been an easy road by any means. However;

> at this point, we are seeing major improvement and we are taking one day at a time.
>
> Mi Mi Diana (grandmother)

Even Health Services gave us a routine call later. They said that Charlie's strain of salmonella was usually found at Easter time, and this was August. The representative agreed with our theory though about the baby chick. To this day we are still not sure, and that worried me for years.

After a few days, we all got back to our old routine. Everyone was doing well and Charlie was great. I watched him all day while I ran my business out of our garage. Our typical day began; Tony took Chelsea to school, and I would get Charlie moving. I had to start answering the phones at nine in the morning. I had my neighbor Gigi helping since right before Charlie's birth. This gave me a little breather. She was great, especially with Charlie. I would be faxing, giving a bottle to Charlie, and then writing a sticky note with the phone on my ear all at the same time. I'm pretty good at multi-tasking. We would have him in the swing or the bouncy seat sometimes while we tried to get work done. Gigi and I would talk baby talk while we were on hold and be faxing simultaneously. I would feed Charlie and play with him in the middle of all this as well. I would even try to squeeze in some laundry. It was a fun and crazy time.

When I look back, there were several little things or signs that bothered me about Charlie. He would choke very easily when he was less than twelve months old. I remember giving him yogurt with the tiny pieces of fruit in it and he would even choke. I remember talking to Tony and saying that he might have a swallowing problem. My gut was telling me something wasn't right about that. There was even one time he turned blue he was choking so badly. I did the Heimlich maneuver on him and the small piece of fruit shot right out of his mouth. Gigi and I were so scared. I thought it was odd how he choked so easily.

He walked at nine or 10 months and sat up at six months, which was fairly normal. It seemed that as soon as I became concerned about something, Charlie would be right on track developmentally with something else, and I would forget the things that concerned me.

> Autism makes me have more patience. It is not easy to understand him right away. You have to make time to try and understand what he is wanting. I have learned that God made people differently and you can't change that. I have helped my brother by making time to help him understand stuff and having time for his needs instead of mine (like the X-Box). It makes me sad sometimes to see that he can't understand what I am saying.
>
> Chelsea (sister)

He was a content baby. He could be in one spot for a long time and not fuss. This really helped as we worked in the office. He slept through the night for the most part, which was contrary to my daughter. I would brag to everyone how good Charlie played and was quiet. When he woke in the morning he didn't fuss that much either.

When he was about four months old, he had a bad bout of diarrhea and then sores on his bottom. This lasted for about two months. He would be lethargic and weak a lot during this time. His bottom would be so sore and raw it would bleed. We tried every over-the-counter ointment. We would be at the doctor's office it seemed, almost every week. We didn't know why this was happening. It finally resolved itself, and we were "normal" again.

He loved to watch *Sesame Street, Barney*, and Disney videos. He would push the rewind button and rewind certain parts over and over again, watching them several times. Trying to get him to take a nap was tough, however. He would scream and try to force his way out of the room or my arms. This could often last for an hour or so. I would come out of his room exhausted, just trying to put him down.

He didn't exercise much speech. He would grunt or would take our hand and put it on the thing that he was wanting. I was a little concerned, but everyone would always say, "he is a boy; that is normal." People would say that boys aren't social and he would talk when he was ready. I agreed and had heard that before as well, but why wouldn't he even say "Momma" or "Dadda?" I found myself comparing him all the time to my daughter. There was something just not right, but I couldn't put my finger on it.

> I will never forget the day I was holding my Maddie in our pool and she was leaning her forhead against mine. I was singing to her without knowing that I was. When I heard what I was singing, I knew it was true, it was the lyrics, "You're everything I hoped for, everything I need, you are so beautiful to me." Maddie must have sensed this moment because she whispered..." You are the Princess Grandma." Can a moment be better than this?
>
> Janice (Grandma)

Charlie's one-year birthday was fast approaching, and he still wasn't saying much of anything. He would continue to pull your hand onto whatever he was wanting, instead of asking for something. He would grunt or moan trying to get out what he wanted. He could not say "milk." We would try and guess what he was wanting. It was like playing charades constantly. He could not say Mom or Dad at all. I would constantly try to teach him to say "nose," "ear," anything. "Milk" was a word I worked on every day to try and get him to say. When he got to be a year old I was feeling a little sad he wouldn't call me "Mommy" or Tony "Daddy."

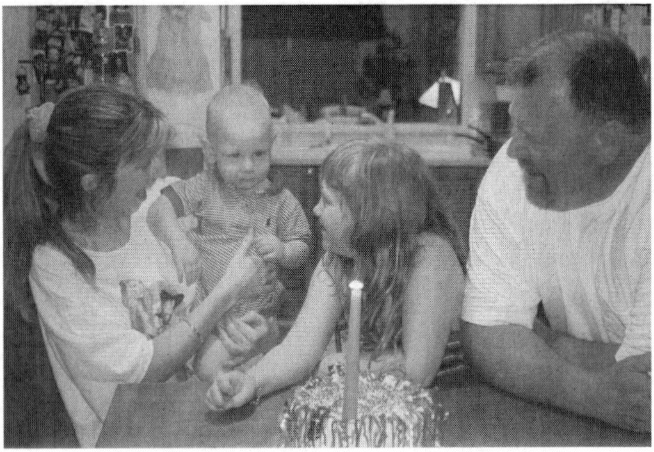

Chelsea, Uncle Bull, and me celebrating Charlie's first birthday 7/11/02

I kept finding myself comparing what Chelsea had done to what Charlie wasn't doing. He started to walk on his toes a lot around six months old. He would hold onto furniture or be in his bouncy seat and always be on his toes. We would make comments on how that must hurt him and how his toenails looked awful. He also would have these strange facial expressions and would just spin in circles aimlessly. When a child is one though you just think, *that's what kids do sometimes*.

Tony had gone to the Internet and looked up autism when Charlie was about one year old because of these things we noticed. After we read the symptoms, we were assured that definitely Charlie didn't have that. They gave the worst scenarios, like head banging, constant tantrums, and rocking back and forth. He did have odd eye movements, and would look at us in the eyes less and less. If he did look at us, it would be at our lips or mouth and not our eyes, even if we told him to look at our eyes. When I would talk to him or ask him something, I could tell that he had no idea what I was saying and would become frustrated. He had a spacey look on his face and would start having a tantrum if I really pressed him on things. We knew he could hear because if he had his back turned, and we called his name, he would turn around. Also, when a plane flew over our house, he would look up.

> I have an eight year old son with autism. Through my son Joseph's autism I have met wonderful people I would have otherwise never met. While I do have a typical child also, (nine-year-old girl, Katie) and I do appreciate all her milestones and all of her accomplishments, there is nothing as wonderful as the feeling you get when your child with autism accomplishes something.
>
> Theresa (mother)

Our primary doctor recommended that Charlie see a speech therapist when he turned two. He didn't make a big deal of it. We chose not to do this because we had heard horror stories about speech therapists only teaching sign language to children. I wanted him to talk and not to rely on sign language. Others kept reminding us that boys often tend to be late talkers. I heard, "he is fine" also. I regret not doing speech therapy earlier and not listening to my gut tell me something was just not right with Charlie.

I waited almost a year (he was two years, 10 months old) and then decided that we actually should get a speech consultation. I assumed we would get the evaluation and that they could then teach me how to help him start to talk. My main focus was really to learn what I needed to do, so that I could help my son. I felt perhaps that I was not doing something I should or that he needed more socialization. My motivation, besides not wanting to see him frustrated, was to catch him up before he got further behind. I had hoped it would be a "quick fix," but my gut was telling me something was just not right.

I called one of the therapists that we used through our home-therapy business. She was wonderful. She came over to the house on a Saturday morning in late May of 2004. She brought all kinds of toys with her to use to evaluate Charlie. All I told her was that I needed help getting him to speak. I also told her he was also getting so frustrated when he would try to tell me something, and we needed some help. I really wasn't nervous about the meeting. My thoughts were to get him jump started. I thought that was all it would take.

> When I first became a special education teacher, I made a conscious choice not to work with

> children with autism. I found the disorder very mysterious and intimidating. At the time, I mistakenly thought there was little or no advancement in working with a child with autism. I could not have been more wrong. My first five years as a teacher, I worked with a few students with autism and then went to learn about a teaching technique called applied behavior analysis (ABA).
>
> Tracy (teacher)

The therapist started by showing Charlie flash cards of different pictures. He got very upset and threw himself on the floor. Charlie would not even look at them for her. Then I noticed he kept walking on his toes while she was trying to engage him. She then used a whistle and some bubbles. He did attempt to blow the bubbles but could not quite get the blowing part. He would blow with his mouth almost shut. She then blew the whistle to show him how use it, but he did not like that either. He held his hands over his ears and cried because of the noise. He would not sit still on the couch for her. The more she tried to do with him the more upset he became.

I knew this was how he operated, but to sit back and watch it was heart breaking. I was doing all that I could not to cry right there. Tony was there and didn't say much either. We tried to observe and just let her do her job. It was obvious that the therapist was having a difficult time trying to complete her tests. My husband then spoke up and said that he had looked up information on autism. She quickly interrupted and said, "I am so glad you said that." I was shocked by her response. Then she asked us a lot of questions, like: "Does he get upset when you change routines? Does he do any rocking? Does he play by himself? Does he line things up over and over again? Does he get upset when you mess up his blocks that are in a row?"

I knew what she was doing. She felt he might be in the autism spectrum, but was asking more questions of us to get a better understanding if this might be the problem.

The therapist recommended that we go and see a pediatric neurologist for further testing. She never actually said. "I think he might have autism," but we knew what the look in her eyes was saying. My stomach was sick. How could this be? It couldn't be this. I remember thinking that I didn't even really understand what autism meant.

> As the father of my own 12-year-old son with autism, whom I also often characterize as being "wired differently." My son has a unique way of describing a beautiful sunset: a "sun rainbow."
>
> Frank (father)

She concluded her evaluation, and Tony and I just walked around stunned. We didn't say too much, because until we saw the doctor we wouldn't know for sure. I felt so sad that day. I didn't know how to absorb all of this. What does this mean?

The next day, I received her evaluation over my work fax. The first page reiterated our concerns about Charlie. I continued on to the oral motor evaluation section. She had administered the Preschool Language Scale test. I looked down on the page and read these words: "Receptive score is 50, percentile is one percent, age equivalent is five months. Expressive score is 61, percentile is one percent, age equivalent is seven months." Tears started streaming down my face and I kept thinking. *He is not five months or seven months; he is almost three years old.* I knew that he needed help but it couldn't be *that* bad. The report also stated he had a severe receptive and expressive delay. *This couldn't be happening*, I thought. *He just needs a little help and he will be fine.*

We called our primary doctor right away to get a referral for a pediatric neurologist. Dr. Martell questioned why we would need this, and we explained the speech evaluation. We faxed over her findings. He didn't think he had autism, but he gave us the referral. Even though I didn't want to believe anything was wrong, my gut was telling me something was just not right.

> Brandon was born in November of 1999, just a couple of days after Thanksgiving. Little did I know that this would be a turning point in my life. As a first-time mom, I knew that there would be challenges, but the challenges that I faced somehow seemed to be different from the ones that other first time moms were going through. This was evident from the first time I saw my child and then started comparing him to other children his age. Even his newborn picture was different. His bright blue eyes wide open, his reddish hair, and his hands tightly closed into fists, so tight that you could see the colors of his knuckles change to white.
>
> Brandon's mom (mother)

> We have, however, learned a newfound respect

for parenting. Had we had a typical child, we might have been the type of people to raise an eyebrow to a child having a meltdown in a department store, but now we understand that many children just can't help it; they have a problem.

Jennifer (mother)

I have a cousin with autism, and having her in my life has been a real blessing and has also led me in the direction of special education. I now have both my BS and MA in early childhood, special education and have been working in the field of autism for many years.

Stephanie (cousin)

My four-year-old son, Garrett, was diagnosed with autism at two and a half. It took some persistence with the doctors, but we thankfully got an early diagnosis. This is the key to the best success in treatment.

Wendy (mom)

I have a son who is now 12 going on 13-years-old who has aspergers. It has been a challenge and a blessing to have him. He was born relatively normal, so I thought, until he hit four years old and he was misdiagnosed with sensory disorder. We went to doctors and therapy and they treated him for it. When my son Zak was in the third grade he was obviously having problems with outburst and meltdowns. It took some one in the school system to tell us he may have autism. Boy what a relief. I knew Zak was different but now we knew what it was.

Sherri (mom)

I teach first grade at a public school in the San Diego area. For the past years, I have had children with autism in my general education classroom. I always begin the year talking about everyone's similarities and differences. We discuss how boring life would be if we were all exactly the same. Our needs and ability to learn are just as different as each and every one of us. By instilling an understanding of those different needs, the children embrace special services or treatments that others may get. My students become very observant and learn techniques that help autistic children cope and communicate.

Denise (teacher)

I have two sons, ages 10 and 3. My older son has aspergers. I also happen to be a psychotherapist, and I had to push to get him the right evaluations to be diagnosed correctly. Moms know when something isn't right, no matter what the professionals sometimes say! It has often been a struggle helping others to understand our son. Alex is so intelligent and observant; he notices minute details that others overlook. Seeing things through his eyes has been a gift. He is honest, even when social norms say he shouldn't be. I wish everyone could see him the way we do!

Michelle (mom)

Having an autistic child has made me realize how important family is. Without the support of my family, I'd probably be depressed knowing my child has something that I can't take away, no matter how hard I try. I've been able to see the good side of autism, and know that I was gifted with a special needs child.

Marlee (mother)

THE DAY EVERYTHING CHANGED

My voice rises to God, and I will cry aloud; My voice rises to God, and he will hear me. In the day of my trouble I sought the Lord.
Psalm 77: 1–2A (NAS)

Early diagnosis was the key for my son. He now has every chance at being great at something.

Debbie (mom)

It was a sunny and bright morning, typical for Fort Lauderdale in June. My husband Tony, my son Charlie, and I were on our way to see Dr. H. He was a pediatric neurologist in the area that was referred to us by our primary doctor. About a month had passed since Charlie had that private speech evaluation. The first appointment we could get for a neurologist was about a month later and here we were. It took 45 minutes just to get to his office through all the morning traffic. I didn't say much to my husband, but I was nervous about what the doctor might say to us.

We walked in the waiting room and signed in our son.

About 15 minutes later the doctor came out and called us back to his personal office. He introduced himself and acknowledged that he had received a report from our private speech therapist and that he understood we were worried about his development. The doctor walked over to the light switch and turned it off. Immediately Charlie went over and turned it back on. I thought that was strange. Why did he do that? Did the doctor purposely do that? The doctor then tried to measure his head circumference, but Charlie would not allow it. Charlie pushed him away and used his grunting noises to try to communicate. Dr. H. then took a pad of paper and said, "Charlie can you draw a circle for me?" Charlie did take the pen and drew a pretty wobbly circle. The last procedure he did was a reflex test, and Charlie allowed him to do that. Dr. H. tapped his knee and arm, and Charlie showed a good reflex move. This took, at the most, a total of three to five minutes.

Dr. H. then sat down behind his desk and said these words, "Your child has Autism Spectrum Disorder. There are severe, moderate, and mild forms. He has the moderate form. We don't know how he got this, and there is no cure either. You will need to get him an MRI, EEG, and a full blood screening for Fragile X, to rule out any physical problems. You will also need to contact your school system to get him some therapy. Here is a prescription for physical, occupational, and speech therapy. Call Plantation General Hospital to get those tests done and I will see you in six weeks."

While he said these shocking words, he had written all of the prescriptions. I was stunned, speechless, and trying not to cry. My head was just spinning. I was feeling dizzy, nauseas, and confused. I felt my world crumbling before my eyes just because of these words from this doctor. I looked at my son that moment and he was oblivious to what this doctor was saying about him. He just kept taking his toy car and moving it back and forth on the floor over and over again. Tony started asking the doctor, "Will he be able to go to school?" The doctor replied, "We don't know. They are doing lots of studies but we don't know what the future holds for 'these kids.' The doctor concluded the appointment, and before we were even out the door, he was dictating the visit in his recorder, "Charles Myers, two years 11 months, diagnosis of autism spectrum disorder, referred for further testing ..."

> Autism has been a blessing in my life in that it has shown me a whole new side of humanity. My brother's life is a life stripped of the complications that a fully functioning brain brings, and, in that, I see how much kindness, gentleness, and most importantly, love, still shines through abundantly.
>
> Seth (brother)

We were numb. Tony and I kept asking each other questions, trying to grasp what the doctor had just said. I didn't fully understand what autism was yet. I just knew of the really extreme cases; like in the movie *Rain Man* in which the man was institutionalized and how he acted and talked really different than others. I remember how smart he was with numbers. We just kept asking each other questions about the comments Dr. H. made. We were so surprised that he just gave a diagnosis so fast. I thought for sure, that he might suspect this diagnosis, but would want to do some tests first. No. Instead, in a matter of less than five minutes, he was telling us that our son has this incurable, neurological disorder. Just get him some therapy and good luck to you. We were not even in his office more than 10 minutes! Then I just felt anger. *How could he tell me my son has Autism after seeing him for five minutes?*

We drove to our primary doctor's office to work on getting the insurance approval for the prescribed procedures. Upon arriving, my husband got out of the car to give the prescriptions to our primary doctor, and I stayed in the car with Charlie. I sat there staring at the note the doctor wrote for the therapists about Charlie. I read it over and over, "autism spectrum disorder 6/28/04." I will have those words in my thoughts forever. I started to cry, well, more like sob. Tony returned and he was crying too. What do you do? Where do you go*? God why*? *Did I do something wrong when I was pregnant*? *Did I eat something wrong to make him like this? Why us?* My mind was racing through my pregnancy, everything I did, ate, and breathed. I kept repeating to myself, *make me sick God, not my child. Maybe the doctor doesn't know what he is talking about. God I am not strong enough to handle this.* These were just some of the frantic thoughts I had that day and days to follow.

We quickly returned to work. Our small home business needed our attention. We had to jump right into dealing with work issues. I was on auto pilot. I worked, but I don't remember much about that afternoon. I do remember, around six that evening, I finished my work and went right into the bathtub to relax. I know that I sat in there for a good hour and had a long cry. I felt like the Charlie I knew prior to ten o'clock that morning was no longer living. I literally felt like that boy died and now I have a new boy. I felt such grief. My heart literally ached for my boy and what his future would hold. I felt guilty for even having these thoughts.

> I have a 12-year-old son that was diagnosed with PDD/NOS at the age of seven. He had been in early intervention programs since he was three to help him with his disability. My husband and I thought he was confused at the beginning since we are both from different countries, he is from Brazil and I am from Nicaragua. There were three languages spoken within both families. We have had ups and downs from asking ourselves why us to how blessed we are to a God for giving us a healthy, happy child.
>
> Matha (mother)

We did not mention anything to our daughter Chelsea who was almost eight. I told my husband, "I don't want *anyone* knowing this until we find out more information." I wanted to wait until the hospital tests were complete. Maybe he had a tumor in his brain? I never thought I would pray for my son to have a tumor. I felt that a tumor was something that could be treated. This was invisible and untouchable. I began praying constantly for my son. I prayed for my husband and my daughter. The two questions that went through my mind the most that next month were, *Will he ever understand who Jesus is and will he ever understand love*? Those two things haunted my thoughts.

We quickly made an appointment at Plantation General Hospital for his MRI and EEG tests. We were told that he could not eat anything after ten the evening before and nothing in the morning (including milk). We arrived at the hospital at eight that morning. My stomach was in shambles about everything then. It had been a week or so since the day we received the diagnosis. After 45 minutes, they called us back. They gave Charlie a drink to make him woozy but not asleep. The nurse needed him to be awake so they could get an accurate reading for the EEG. Most things were scary to Charlie, and he became agitated very easily. He would grunt, trying to communicate his fears. The nurse, Tony, and I had to hold him down while he screamed and we tried to get the liquid medicine in his mouth to help him go to sleep. We waited 30 to 45 minutes for it to work. It didn't. The nurse then said that we should try a little more, so we went through this again, holding him down. It took all three of us and we were still barely able to do this. To watch my son being held down by three adults and see the fear in his eyes was almost more than I could handle. My stress level was at its highest. Another 30 minutes or so went by and he was groggy but awake and still agitated. My nerves were shot. I was so anxious and worried about my son. Then the nurse tells us that some kids just don't get groggy enough to do this. I felt like punching her lights out. *What do you mean?* Could she have told us this earlier so we could make other arrangements? We had wasted three hours and put our son through unnecessary torture. We were unable to do the tests. We left that hospital, and never wanted to return again. Charlie didn't go to sleep until ten that evening and suffered from diarrhea all evening. It was a day I will never forget.

> That which we were able to block out became the very thing that turned his world upside down. It made the relationship between my husband and I (and God) grow to the point where I

> knew no matter what happened we would not see it alone. We have a picture now that I never thought would be a part of our album. It is a picture of Vincent on the Homecoming court representing the Sophomore class.
>
> Mrs. G. (mom)

Meanwhile my sister Kelly and her family had arrived from Arizona to visit with us that second week in July (just two weeks after the diagnosis). I begged Tony not to say a word. I was really fearful also that if we told anyone, they would treat him differently. I didn't want that. Charlie was in his prime that week. I felt like this big light was flashing on him the entire time saying, "I have autism." For instance, one night we went out to eat and he kept staring up at the fans and making strange eye movements. I was so scared that my family would notice and figure it out. Anytime someone tried to talk to him, we would say that he was shy. He would never respond, but he was good at giving high fives so we did that constantly to show that he was somewhat engaged. My sister, my brother, and their families all came over to our house for dinner. This was the same day as when we tried to do the EEG and MRI tests and wasted the whole morning. Kelly and her family were going back home the next morning.

We were all at the table, except for my mom, and I felt like the time had come to tell my family about what had been going on. All of a sudden, and in the middle of a conversation I said, "I need to tell you all something." They all looked at me with scared expressions, and then my sister said, "You're not pregnant are you?" We all laughed and then all I could say was, "It's about Charlie." I started to cry.

My husband, Tony, looked at me with tears in his eyes and said, "It is okay." Tony quickly told them that Charlie was okay, because everyone had a terrified look on their faces. Tony went on to explain that we had been at the hospital all morning, and that Charlie had been diagnosed with autism just a little over a week before. I was a mess. I was tired, depressed, and exhausted from keeping this all in. My sister Kelly prayed for us right away which made me feel a lot better. I felt I had their support now even though I had no idea what was in store for us. They also all said, in their own way that they had some suspicions that something wasn't right. I needed my brother's support so badly, and that night, I knew I had it with his hugs. The night ended on a happy note, and we had a birthday cake for Charlie and his sister Chelsea. He turned three and she turned nine just a day apart.

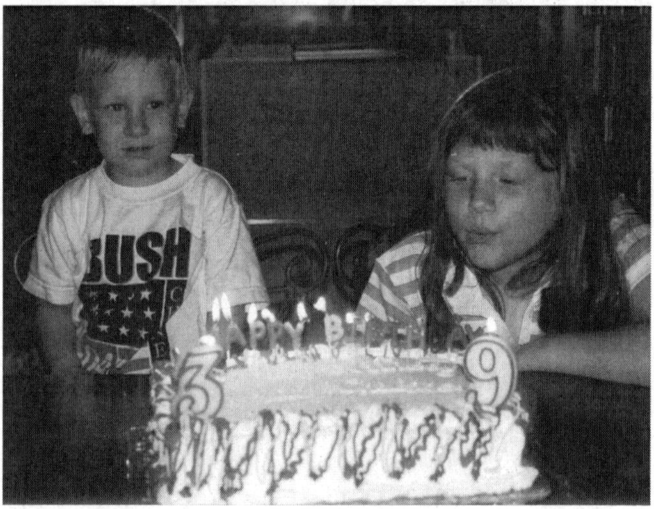

Celebrating with family on Chelsea's 9th and Charlie's 3rd birthday, just days after we received the diagnosis.

My family left and I felt some relief that I was able to get it all out. I started to think again about the day we had at the hospital. I felt the hospital diagnostic center employees were very incompetent and had no training with autism. The next morning, I began calling other places that could perform the tests that Charlie needed. I called Joe Dimaggio's Children's Hospital in Hollywood. This was about 30 minutes away from where we lived. I explained to the nurse our experience and asked if there was something else that could be administered to him to make him groggy. She explained that there was and gave us some better advice also to help prepare and to help him relax before the tests. I scheduled the tests with them in another two weeks. That was the earliest they had. We were ready for round two.

> My little girl is my hero. She has come a long way from her nonverbal days. She is happy to see me. She tells me she loves me all the time. It is so refreshing to have someone around that is almost always happy. She doesn't worry about all the nonsense around her. There are certain things that she likes to do and there are other things she could care less about. She loves to play video games and eat...as long as she can be doing both of those she is happy, the simple life...normal children worry about too much nonsense and follow what everyone else does regardless if it is wrong or right. My daughter just does what she wants to do...no peer pressure. We love her so much!
>
> Liz (mother)

In the meantime we asked our primary doctor if he could give us a doctor's referral for a second opinion from another neurologist. We wanted affirmation on Charlie's diagnosis. We felt like the first doctor didn't really do a full assessment. Tony and I wanted to be sure of the diagnosis before he was "labeled" autistic. Our appointment was on August 16, 2004 almost two months from the first diagnosis we had received. I was anxious and curious to see what this doctor would say. This neurologist was a female, and the other doctor was a male. I was really hoping she wouldn't think he had autism. She had us in her office/examination room for over 45 minutes, and she watched Charlie's every move. She was very thorough with her questions. She even tried to assess Charlie's heart rate but he was screaming and flopping on the floor, so she could not get those vitals. I felt very confident in her examination. We explained to her our problems trying to get the MRI and EEG, and she informed us that she wouldn't recommend they be done. I was shocked. She said their results wouldn't change anything, and putting him through them would be a very difficult ordeal. She also wanted to administer a medication to calm him. She was doing her own study of it, and it was a medication given to Alzheimer's patients. We said a quick "no way" to the medication. At that time, he wasn't out of control with his behavior, and I didn't want him on any medication unless he was uncontrollable or too uncomfortable. I was more worried about the side effects and long term problems that come with some medications.

At the conclusion of the visit, she said, "I do believe he is on the autism spectrum." Until she uttered those words, I still felt there was hope that something else was going on. It was really awful, again, I was actually praying for a brain tumor or something we could see on an x-ray and could try and fix. The nail was in the coffin. Even though, in my heart, I knew he had this disorder, I was still hoping she would see something else instead of autism. I walked ahead of Tony to the car and just cried and cried. I was a mess. I think back on that day, and it was much tougher than the first day we received this diagnosis. She had given us more hope and explained much more to us about autism, but she gave us the reality of what might be in his future. I got to our home office and felt like I was in a fog. It was one of the worst days of my life.

> I am a grandmother of two autistic children, this may sound contradictory, but the joy and happiness I receive by knowing these two little people is without description.
>
> Thelma (grandmother)

The day came, and here we were ready to make our second attempt at getting the MRI and EEG done. We decided to try one more time at getting these tests done for Charlie, to rule out any physical problems he might have, despite the second doctor's opinion. The nurse asked us to keep him up as late as possible the night before and wake him up as early as possible in the morning. Tony and I stayed up with him until about one o'clock in the morning and then Tony woke him up at five in the morning. We headed out again to Joe Dimaggio's Children's Hospital. It took 30 minutes to check us in, and Charlie was very agitated, hungry, cranky, and probably sleepy too.

I went back to registration by myself while Tony stayed with Charlie in the waiting area. I gave them all my insurance information and then the lady informed us that our appointment was rescheduled due to an insurance matter. I felt the heat rising to my face. "What do you mean insurance matter?" I said. She explained that they had not received the proper authorization yet, and that the neurologist's office should have let us know. I was so upset. I said, "I have the appointment with you all, not my doctor's office; It is your responsibility to let us know."

She said, "There is nothing we can do." Tony and I marched to the administrative offices and made a complaint. They took us back to registration and tried to resolve this over the phone with our doctor's office.

Meanwhile Charlie hadn't eaten or drank anything for over twelve hours and had only slept for approximately four hours. Imagine a three year old in that predicament. He was screaming and flopping on the hospital floors. For the first time, I was glad to see this display. I wanted them to see what they had done to him since they were trying to send us home. Tony dealt with the hospital staff while I tried to hold down Charlie in the hospital hallway. I couldn't control him. People were now paying attention because he was screaming so loudly. A nice lady came up to him and asked if he wanted a sticker and that just made it worse. I wanted to crawl in a corner and cry. They finally came out and apologized and said that they would reschedule today's appointment. I didn't know what to do. Was God saying he shouldn't have these tests? Were we doing the right thing for our son? Why were we having all these obstacles?

> We have an angel living amongst us. We are strong in our faith, but by no means holier than thou. Drew, on the other hand seems to be drawn to all things good and spiritual. Besides the fact that he loves to be in church and does

> his version of singing praise to God, he loves the Bible and pictures of Jesus or Mary. He has the sweetest demeanor and best smile that just lights up the room.
>
> Megan (mother)

We scheduled another appointment for a couple weeks later. This was now the last week of August 2004. I told my husband that I could not bear to go again, so I asked my mom if she would go with Tony for the third attempt at getting the MRI and EEG. My mom supported Tony while I stayed and ran the office. My emotional state, at this point, was so fragile. I just couldn't watch him scream and not be able to tell us what he wanted. Charlie was a trooper and did well. He got upset a little bit, but not too extreme. They were able to get both tests completed. When Tony pulled up to the house, Charlie was fast asleep in his car seat. He had that gooey stuff in his hair from doing the EEG test. I was so glad that was over for him. Mom had been such a tremendous help by doing that for me.

That summer of 2004 was a blur. One day, I was a mess, depressed, and crying all day. The next day, Tony was having a tough time. It seemed as though we took turns for each other. I remember telling him once to be patient with me. I said, "Let me just be sad for a little while." We both went to book stores and grabbed practically everything on the shelves about autism, which wasn't much. I read books every night and cried as I read them. Most books described exactly how Charlie had been acting. I kept being reminded that he did have this disorder with every book I read. For instance, I was reading one book that mentioned a mother who was feeling like her child had died. When I read that, I literally gasped to myself. I had felt that but had never told anyone of my feelings. Those two months, July and August, were my deep grieving time. I felt the son I had prior to June 28 was one child, and on June 29, I was given another child. I cried for my "new" son, and I cried because the dreams that I had for him might not come true. Tony and I thought we were traveling on this certain road, and then God said, "no you are going to go this way instead. It is a little rockier but this is the path for you." It was extremely scary.

> I promised myself when I found out that my daughter, my oldest child, had autism that she would never see me unhappy, angry, or sad. I believe that a parent's personality defines a child's outlook and eventual personality. By the time my son was diagnosed, he was already in such a loving environment that it rubbed off on him. I could never in my wildest dreams have asked for such loving and giving children. Yes, it has been difficult and trying at time, and sometimes still is, but if you can hang in there as a parent, the unconditional love these little people give you can never be measured. I am the proudest parent around.
>
> Gabi (mother)

When a parent gets a diagnosis from a doctor, whether it is autism, cerebral palsy, cancer, down syndrome, diabetes, asthma, or anything for that matter, you will question everything. That is what we did for a good two months. The big question of course is "why?" What plan does God have for us? I was always told when I was growing up, that God uses our tough life experiences for his good. I wondered how this could be good. How can a child who can't speak, be good? How can a child who looks scared so often, be good? How can a child who can't tell you something hurts, be good? How can a child that won't look you in the eyes, be good? How can a child who hits himself when he's frustrated, be good? I read and read the Bible and searched for why this was happening to our family. Why was God using us? Up to this point in my life, I had felt that God had already used me enough in my 37 years.

I was feeling insecure about being able to help my son. Would I be able to give him what he needs? I struggled to find the good in this diagnosis. I remember someone coming up to me when I was in this fog and telling me that this autism will be a blessing and that Charlie would show me so many things. I thought, *autism a blessing, I don't think so.* I got really angry at the comment. I thought there was no way they could have any idea how bad this is right now. None of this could possibly be a blessing.

Later, as you read on, you will see how God uses Charlie to show me and my family so many things. One of the best parts is how he brings our family even closer. God never wastes a hurt.

> When my first grand-daughter, Madison, was diagnosed with autism, I literally felt that I could not breathe. I was furious with my son for having her tested. It was better to be able to make believe than endure this diagnosis. I knew for a long time that things were not right but I did not want it to be confirmed. I could not bear the pain on my son's face and would have liked to fall asleep and not wake up, maybe

forever. After our family found a variety of ways to communicate without using this word "autism" and bolstering each other to rise above this "temporary" situation, we started to breathe again.

Janice from Brooklyn (grandma)

My son's autism was the catalyst that took us away from our business that was consuming our whole life. It made me realize how important family is.

Joe (dad)

I still remember my time in the womb after sixteen years. Almost like that, I recognized my existence in that bubble. Then, coming out into the world was such a big scare. From the dark I came into the light. Is it any wonder we cry upon entry? Then, only several years later would my parents discover that I had been afflicted with asperger's syndrome, a special, milder form of autism that could be dubbed the "genius syndrome." Its sufferers become extremely bright, precocious children but are still confined in a certain sense into their own world. I would not discover this information until I was in the school system many years later.

Vince (16 year old living with aspergers)

To all the moms out there who arrange their schedules around their child's rigid routine so that they can have a peace of mind, and to all the parents who don't know about it. If you can't have a sense of humor of the trials and tribulations then you will burn out and be of no use to your child. I give kudos to all of those parents too.

Damarius (mother)

As parents of children with autism, we cross all races and nationalities. We're rich and poor, single parents and married couples, conservatives and liberals. Some of us are shy, others are loud. Just about anyone can be inducted in to our club. In twenty minutes, there will be a new initiation. That is how often a parent hears "Your child has autism.". This year doctors will say that 24,000 times. That is a lot of parents who know just what I am talking about.

Amy (mother)

I am a second-time-around parent of a duly diagnosed 11-year-old child and a duly diagnosed eight-year-old child. I have adopted both girls. I adopted their birthmother when she was ten and a half years old; at 11 she was diagnosed with onset schizophrenia. With the background out of the way I will tell you about my 11-year-old angel girl, Christy. Christy was diagnosed as autistic when she was two. She mostly speaks in echolalia (echoing). She is low functioning. Due to lots of behaviors (destruction, aggression, and not sleeping) I had to place her in a behavioral residential setting. I still see her weekly. The blessing of Christy is that God chose to give her to me.

Linda (adoptive mother)

We have been blessed with an amazing team of therapists and teachers who have worked wonders for Matthew and provided tremendous support to our family. Dealing with autism is never easy, but it has brought us so much in these last two years. Mostly, it has given me a new perspective: greater compassion, patience, understanding, and an appreciation for what truly matters in life. The best blessing of all though, is that I have gained a true understanding of my value as a mother, not only of two boys, but two perfect boys.

Emily (mother)

YOUR CHILD HAS AUTISM, NOW WHAT?

For I know the plans I have for you, declares the Lord... plans to prosper you and not to harm you, plans to give you hope and a future. Jeremiah 29:11 (NIV)

Our 'lil man' is now speaking thanks to the help of a wonderful speech pathologist which he sees three times a week. The sensory issues he has are being worked on by his physical therapist. Don't let anyone tell you when you feel something is not right you are wrong. God only knows where we would be right now if we had continued listening to Corey's first doctor.

Peggy (step-mom)

It had been a difficult road so far. Some days I didn't want to talk about autism and other days I wanted to cry about it. My family and friends were really supportive. I dealt with my grief each day differently. The first thing I had to learn to accept was that he had autism. The next step I took was to replace the picture I had of my son the way I thought he was, and replace it with a new picture. I had to look at him in a different light, which was a big step. I often tell people; before you found out your child had autism you were traveling down a road going north, and then when you found out he had autism, you seemed to make a sharp right. It is just a different path than you expected to go. It might even take longer to get to the destination, but hopefully, you will end up at the same spot no matter which way you travel.

I really got through that first year by prayer and support of my family and friends. I also did research practically everyday. I read books, I went on the internet, and I spoke to other mothers of children with autism. I think that speaking with other mothers or fathers of children with autism was the most valuable to me. These people had gone through what I had already. I remember my friend Claudia giving me the name of a lady she knew that had a son with autism who was in his thirties or so. It took me almost two months to call her, but I finally did. She gave me so much encouragement. Her son was severely affected and now he is married with children running his own computer consulting business. At the end of the conversation, I asked her if I could call her son because I had just had two different computer repairmen trying to fix our office computers. They each charged $100 an hour, worked for several hours each, and could never fix it. He ended up coming over (driving about an hour to my house) and was able to fix my computer. I then asked him what I owed him for the services and he said, "I don't know, maybe $25.00?" He explained how his wife did all the finances. He just seemed to be a shy person, but was able to talk to me briefly about how he felt when he was younger and how he got through. I told him to wait a minute while I go get my checkbook. I came back and gave him $100 an hour just like the other guys charged. When he saw the amount written, his eyes got real big. I told him, "You charge $100 an hour because that is the going rate. The other guys couldn't even fix it and you did." He just smiled and went on his way. That day was a pivotal day in my journey. I knew that day that Charlie would be alright. I knew it wouldn't be an easy journey, but I knew at that point, we would be okay.

> My son reminds me daily of an overseas trip promised when he turns 21 to go to London. My son is exceedingly polite, but is sometimes inclined to inappropriately verbalize thoughts, for example, about the size of a patron entering a store or restaurant: "look at the big, fat... ." His older sisters usually tackle him, cover his mouth, and gently wrestle him out of the establishment, all of us struggling to control our laughter, so we can address the impolite comment.
>
> Frank (dad)

For me, finding out what this autism was, and how to help my son was key. After I grasped the enormity of it and what plan we were going to take, I started to lift out of my depression. I first had to figure out what issues Charlie had. What problems was Charlie struggling with? What was Charlie behind in? Once I knew the answers to those questions, then I searched out different ways I could help him with these specific things. We still would have our tough days, but they seemed to be fewer.

I know when we were told the first time we were in shock. The hardest part of this diagnosis for me, was hearing; "I don't know how he got this," and "It is not curable."

It cuts like a knife. The only information the doctor gave us was to go to our school district and get an evaluation. He gave us prescriptions for therapy, but who were we to call, where were we to go? We had to do all the leg work and figure out how to tackle this autism. Here are some suggestions of where you need to begin that have helped our family:

1. *Do your own evaluation.* You need to look at a few specific areas. The traits that are affected with autism are social, cognitive-receptive language (understanding what you are saying), and communication. If any of these areas are not where they should be then you should talk to the doctor about your concerns. Don't listen to someone say, "Oh he is just a boy and they develop slower." The more quickly you identify the problem, the better the outcome can be. As a relative or caregiver, you have a gut instinct if something is not right with your child/grandchild. Go with that feeling and get answers. The worst thing that can happen is your child gets some therapy and testing when it wasn't needed. It can't hurt your child.

Autism spectrum disorder has an array of symptoms. For example, your child may play with a toy in an atypical way. For instance, Charlie will play with a car by laying down on the floor and moving the tires back and forth, back and forth. He would just stare for an hour at the wheels moving back and forth. He would not play with the toy or make car noises as typical little boys do. A typical child will have imaginary play and use the toy appropriately. He would always line things up, like blocks, cars, and trains. If you took one out of order, he would get very upset. This is a child with autism's way of soothing himself and feeling less anxious. They are making order out of their mixed up world.

> I have taken on the "mission" of delivering a message to those who do not understand this difference in the children that have been recognized as having autism. To the people in McDonalds watching me struggle with my child (because a 20 minute line up is a little too long to endure even for a "normal" three year old) with an expectation for me to "control" my child because he is freaking out and running away...please understand that what you see is a tiny glimpse of what a parent of an autistic child may go through.
>
> Damarius (mother)

I would ask Charlie simple questions, and he would look spacey and not understand what I was asking him. He would never have great eye contact. It would be very fleeting. He loved to take pictures though and loved to stare at the flash that would come on. He always seemed "in his own world." We just took it that he wasn't interested in what we were saying or doing.

Charlie would cover his ears a lot. His ears were and are very sensitive to sounds. One time he kept saying "zero." I had no idea what he was talking about. We were playing a game on the television. I said, "You want the TV off?" Then I turned the game off, and he got really upset. I kept trying to guess what was wrong, and he kept saying "zero." Then I turned the volume down, because by then he was screaming so loudly, and he calmed down immediately. I noticed the volume on the screen has a scale of 0 - 10. He was trying to tell me to turn it down to zero even though it had only been on two or three.

He goes back and forth of pulling on all his tags in his clothes. He will do this for months and then just stop. A few months later he starts again. Charlie would chew on his shirts so hard that he would put holes in them. They would be soaked from his sucking on them so much. It was his way of calming himself down. His sensory system was out of sorts. He needed to feel that deep pressure in his mouth.

He loves to be squeezed when he gets really upset. It also calms him. We even invested in a bean bag chair. We would put him on the bed and then the bean bag on top of him (over his belly and legs) and gently put pressure on him. He loved that and would always say "gen, gen" (meaning again, again).

If we changed routines sometimes he would get upset. If he watched a program every morning at 10am and then one day I put it on something else, he would get upset and grunt. He walks on his toes still when he is bare foot or just in socks. He uses a lot of echolalia speech, which is when he repeats back what I say. I might say, "Charlie, say good-bye." and he will say, "Charlie, say good-bye." Or I might say, "Charlie, give them a hug" and he might say, "Charlie, give them a hug."

Things to look for at the age of two that would give you some concern include: walking on toes a lot, covering ears a lot, acting like he/she can't hear, not understanding a simple command, having very little speech, not interested in playing with other kids, doesn't even notice when people walk in the room, can stare at something for a long period of time and be content, lines things up and gets upset when you break the order, or has excellent computer skills but can't understand a simple command you give him. These are just some examples you can look for.

> I have a three-year-old autistic child named Darian and he's a handful. On his good days and bad days, I don't give up. I believe in my heart that one day he will snap out of this little world of his and see me. I can't explain how hard it is to not hear your child tell you simple everyday words like, Mommy I love you. I'd give anything to hear my son say that to me at least once.
>
> Marlee (mom)

I remember trying to explain to people what this autism was. My husband would always use the example that Charlie was like a computer with the correct hardware but the software is a little mixed up. We just have to rearrange the software. I always explain that the wires in Charlie's brain have little shorts. Some days the wires seem to be plugged in well and on other days, the wires seem really loose. A key ingredient predicament with my son is that he looks "normal." He has blonde hair, blue eyes, fair skin, and a great smile (I of course am a little biased). He has no outward appearance of having any problems, so that makes it difficult for people to understand why he may act so strange or get upset so easily.

The Autism Society of America has written down some signs of autism. They are the following:

- Spins objects; sustains odd play
- Aloof manner; difficulty mixing with others
- Repetitive movements (hand-flapping, rocking)

- Laughs/cries/shows distress for no clear reason
- Uneven, gross/fine motor skills (may not kick a ball but can stack blocks)
- Severe language deficits
- Difficulty expressing needs; gestures or points instead of speaking
- Not responsive to verbal cues; acts as if deaf
- Echolalia (repeats words instead of responding)
- Insists on sameness; inflexible about routines
- Inappropriate attachment to objects
- Noticeable physical over or under activity

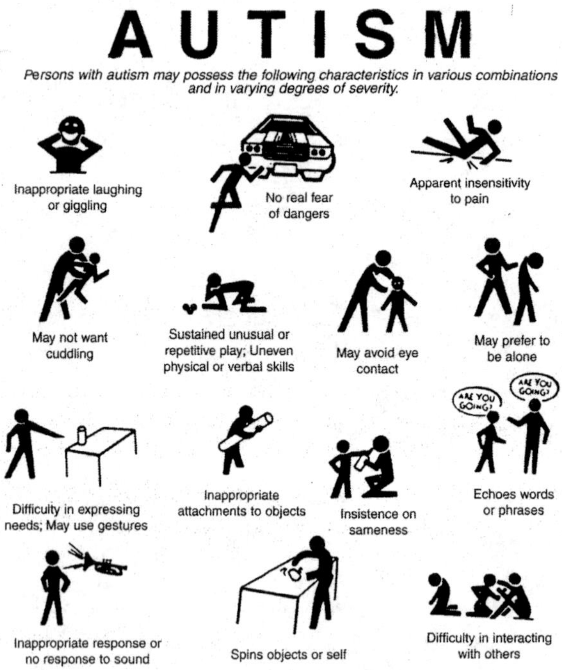
AUTISM
Persons with autism may possess the following characteristics in various combinations and in varying degrees of severity.
Inappropriate laughing or giggling
No real fear of dangers
Apparent insensitivity to pain
May not want cuddling
Sustained unusual or repetitive play; Uneven physical or verbal skills
May avoid eye contact
May prefer to be alone
ARE YOU GOING?
ARE YOU GOING?
Difficulty in expressing needs; May use gestures
Inappropriate attachments to objects
Insistence on sameness
Echoes words or phrases
Inappropriate response or no response to sound
Spins objects or self
Difficulty in interacting with others

Remember, if you see your child with some of these issues,

it would be wise to make an appointment with your family doctor or pediatric neurologist and tell them of your concerns.

2. *Do lots of research.* The Internet has a mound of great information. Step one should be to get a complete understanding of autism. You can't tackle something if you don't understand what you are trying to tackle. Then you should inventory your child's issues. Every child with autism can be so different. One child may have a lot of sensory issues while another may have a lot of communicative issues.

> My son has a very hard time making friends. He also has a hard time academically, he is below grade level. We always encourage him to do his best, and no matter what we are very proud of him. He has a younger sister that is nine and they love each other so much and are very protective of each other.
>
> Matha (mother)

Read as much information about this disorder as you can find. There are so many different opinions and approaches to autism. You need to decide what help you need, so that you can pick the appropriate treatment for your child. Find books to read. There are so many different ideas, and what works for one child may not work for another. There are different diets and medical treatments out there. Many kids have had success on the gluten/casein-free diet. Our family's approach has been so far to try and manage this disorder without any drastic interventions. I am trying to refrain from giving him any medications as possible. I have a fear that they may make him flaccid and not himself. I just don't feel comfortable yet, giving him something that hasn't been studied that long on children. Some kids require medication. I have witnessed stories of families turning to medicine and it made a huge difference in their child. So many of the medications available have a risk of more side effects, than actual benefits that help the problem. This is a personal choice and something you need to discuss with your doctor.

Be very careful of some information given on the Internet. Stay away from things that claim your child can take a pill, and it will *cure* the autism. No such thing exists. You need to do your homework before doing anything drastic. There is *no* simple pill for autism. I know it is tempting to try but it is simply not true. Save your money for therapies or something else your child will truly need. Also, stay away from doctors who promise they can help you but don't take insurance and charge over $500 a visit. I am not sure they are looking out for your child's best interests. The bottom line is that you should do a whole lot of research so that you know what you are up against. Then you can stand up and put on your armor and fight for your child. In chapter nine, I will list many informative resources that I've found to be helpful.

> One thing that I want parents to know is... autism is something you have, not something you are. I think too many times we tend to unfairly label people. I have a one-year-old son, Zackery, who has autism. I used to say I have a son who is autistic. Later I grew to know more about who he is as a person, I began to realize

> that there is so much more to Zackery than just the fact hc has autism.
>
> Esmeralda (mother)

3. *Get speech therapy asap if needed.* My immediate priority for Charlie was to get him to speak. He was three and hardly used any words at all. I felt that his ability to speak would relieve most of his frustrations. Speech is one of the most important things to treat aggressively and immediately.

My son was introduced to the PECS system at the first school he attended. This stands for Picture Exchange Communication System. To this day, I feel it has helped him the most. It is a system that places the picture and the corresponding word on a little square card for the child's reference so he can understand what he is being told. For example, I would say, "Charlie give me the cup." I would be practically touching the cup, but he would look all over and then get frustrated, because he had no idea what I was talking about. I would then show him the picture card of a cup and make him look at it. Then I would point to the cup I wanted, and he would better understand it. It came slowly, but the system worked.

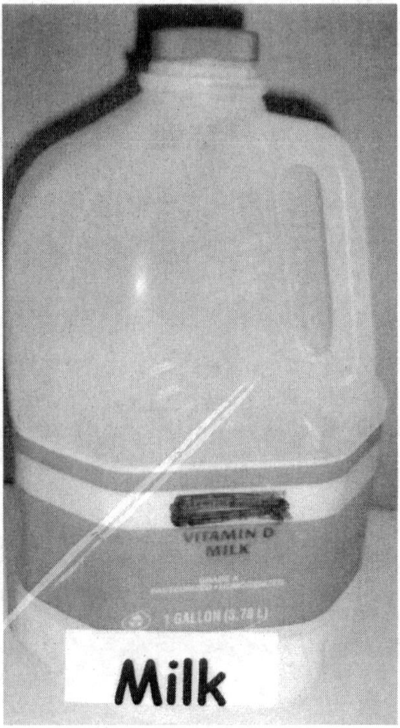

This is an example of the pictures we made ourselves on the computer to help him speak and work on receptive language.

It was only a week after his diagnosis that I took Charlie to his first speech therapist, Jessica. The first week he would not say anything and she tried to teach him sign language to prompt his words. I will never forget the first time he signed the word "*more.*" Tears ran down my face. He didn't verbally say it, but he said it with his hands, and I was happy. A week or so later, he actually said the word "*more.*" Jessica also kept trying to get him to say, "I want ________." One day it just came out. It was hard to understand, but Jessica and I knew exactly what he said. We both had tears in our eyes that day. It was coming, little by little.

> I have a child who has a difference, it is his normal, and all I ask of society is to take into consideration that all of the children who require a label to get help, only need society to see that they have something to learn from them and that, we, as parents are responsible for ensuring that we advocate on their behalf. It is not the same as tolerating bad driving or poor diet. All of which are choices. Choices that we make, we are very well aware (or at least I hope you are) have a direct impact on how our lives "turn out." Children born with a difference, whether it be physical or mental, didn't get a choice and neither did their parents.
>
> Damarius (mother)

4. *Call your school district.* Once you get a diagnosis, call your local school district. There is a government program called Child Find which is covered under the I.D.E.A law which provides a *free and appropriate education* to all children with disabilities. There are two programs, one for children under three and one for children three to five years old. There is an initial evaluation to see if your child even will need such services. After this, they refer you to the separate evalua-

tors, such as speech therapy, occupational therapy, psychologist, hearing tests, and other various tests according to what your child's needs are. Each step can take several weeks to a month to get the appointments and evaluations.

The quicker you can get your child help, the better the outcome can be. This system is sometimes hard to negotiate, but you need to stand firm. There are so many rules and laws to follow, so you may have to take lots of notes and definitely buy yourself a nice big calendar you can carry with you. You know what your child needs, and you should make sure he/she gets it no matter what. You will not make friends with these people. Unfortunately, these agencies have to follow a budget and they look at your child in this manner. You know what your child will need and your focus is only getting your child better. *Stay strong*.

> Vinnie, my son, doesn't ever worry about peer pressure!
>
> Susan (mom)

5. *Go out socially with your child.* Take your child as many places as possible. It is difficult when he/she has tantrums and sensory overload, but the more you do the more they learn to tolerate social settings. I got to a point where I couldn't even go to Target with Charlie. He would have a fit for no reason, and I couldn't physically get him out of the store. I got plenty of looks by people that assumed he was just a spoiled brat. I was never really embarrassed, but I felt overwhelmed when he would do these things.

I remember once I was taking my daughter to her first gymnastics class and Charlie was with us. I had to sign her in, and there were a lot of parents standing in the waiting area watching their children. He would not go in the gym. He was flopping on the floor, screaming as loud as he could. It was just too much stimuli for him. I finally said "bye bye" several times, and he came grudgingly. After that, I just learned to be calm. Sometimes, I would even have to leave my cart full of items in a store because, there was no way I could finish my shopping without making the situation worse.

We live by Disney World and I have to say those parks have helped him a whole lot. The first time he went, all he would do was cry with his hands over his ears. He didn't like to look at any of the characters. He would get very upset. Now we go there and he loves it. He still will cover his ears at times, but when he goes through the entrance he puts his hands in the air and screams, "Yes!" Those parks have so much sensory information for them. It gets them used to doing, hearing, smelling and seeing things all at the same time. He still struggles sometimes but we get through it. We will have to sometimes find a quiet corner somewhere to just calm his nerves. They also have a guest assistance pass you can ask for that is free that helps you get closer to the front of lines because they are unable to wait in 45 minute lines. This has helped us tremendously. Before we knew about this pass we would only be able to do one or two rides because he would get so upset waiting. He has no concept of "we have to wait a few minutes." Most of these parks have these options, you just have to ask and explain how your child has difficulty. Thank you, Disney.

> I am so proud of my daughter Chelsea, she is so patient with her brother and although she will not willingly admit it, she loves him very much. She has been so instrumental in his progress and

> it has been said that GOD gives special kids to special parents. If this is true than I believe that GOD gave Charlie a special sister! She accepts him as he is ..."just Charlie."
>
> Tony (dad)

6. *Key words to use*. One of the best pieces of advice was from Marilee over at CARD. This stands for Center for Autism and Related Disabilities. This is one of the programs funded by government grants located at universities throughout Florida. She made us a card that had Velcro attachments to it. One side said, "FIRST _______." and the other side said, "THEN _____."

This statement is so crucial with kids who have autism. It organizes their thoughts better. I found out later this is a tool they use in behavior analysis. Earlier in his diagnosis we went around the house and took pictures with our digital camera of things that he liked or places we went a lot. For instance we took pictures of the Target store, milk carton, his shoes, cheerios, the car, our church, things like this. After we took them we would write the word of the picture under it and then make small cards and laminate them so they would last. We used these a lot at the beginning to help us communicate with him and to figure out what he wanted. I got to the point and even do this now, usually I can tell by his grumbling language what he wants but I still try and get him to say it or point to the picture of what he wants. We used the pictures that were Velcro on the card that said, "First _____." Then _____." at first, and then we just used our words several months later, and he understood what we were saying. That statement has saved me a lot of tantrums along the way. For example, if I had to go to the grocery just to get milk and have him with me, it could be an hour-long, arduous task if I didn't use these key words. Before I would go to the store I would say, "*First* we need to go get milk, *Then* we will go play on the playground." He will repeat back this statement and then he keeps saying it to himself over and over again. It has worked so well with him, he knows what to expect.

> The same week we found out we were expecting our second child, and three months before our son, Matthew, turned three, we took Matthew to see a pediatric neurologist, who confirmed our worst fears. Matthew's communication difficulties, restricted play patterns, social anxiety, emotional volatility, rigid thinking, and obvious sensory processing problems, when all considered together, presented a clear picture: Matthew was autistic. The excitement of another child on the way, contrasted by the overwhelming grief and fear we faced were such opposing forces, perhaps it was enough to keep us in balance.
>
> Emily (mother)

7. *Sign up with Autism Society groups.* Try and find your local chapter of the Autism Society. It is a great support network and has a wealth of information. It is also helpful to meet other parents and siblings that you can relate and connect with at different points on your journey. There is also a national group called the Autism Society of America. Signing up with these groups will allow you to receive a constant stream of information. I get almost daily emails

from our local chapter. It has not only been a wealth of information but also an encouragement. Thank you Donna Lorman.

> Yes, parenting a child with autism provides the reward of putting life in perspective and access to daily life lessons that would otherwise be unavailable.
>
> Frank (father)

8. *Take a breather.* Take time for yourself. I have been a bad example of this, but it truly is the most important thing you can do to help your child. If you are stressed and exhausted, you are not able to help your child as well and as much as you need to. I find that my quiet time sometimes means getting up 15 to 30 minutes before everyone else. Sometimes, right after both kids leave for school, I take a half hour to walk and organize my thoughts (that is if you aren't working). I am not a morning person but doing this gives me a fresh start. This is my time of prayer and a time of calmness before the day begins.

My husband and I hardly go out on dates because we are apprehensive to leave Charlie with anyone. What if he has a bad tantrum? What if he hurts himself? Can the babysitter handle him? Will he run out the front door and not be noticed? Who can we find who will change his diaper at age six? We have only done this a few times, but I am going to try and do it more often, because it helps him as much as it helps us.

Often kids with autism don't seem to need sleep. We have had this problem off and on with Charlie. For a while, he went through a stage in which he woke up every morning at three and went around opening and slamming doors throughout the house. If you tried to stop him, he would get more upset. That really made me feel exhausted in the morning. Tony and I seem to take turns dealing with things like this.

> When I took my baby home from the hospital, he was always quiet, he never cried but would follow me with his eyes, hands opening and closing rapidly. His pediatrician would always be amazed at how fast he was developing. By the time he was 10 months, he walked and could say things like "clock" and "wheel." He would spin anything he could, tops, wheels, loved to watch the washing machine, pinwheels and he would do it for hours at a time. This is also when he started having tantrums. His tantrums would last up to 30 minutes and without a logical explanation as to what set him off. He would kick, bite, punch, and bang his head on the floor. His face red with anger and his eyes seemed to be fixed, like we were not there at all. This was the part that scared us the most. Then, once he calmed down, he would start laughing, he would blink, and act as if nothing had happened.
>
> Brandon's mom (mother)

9. *Sign up for medwaiver.* It is a program that can cover autism through Developmental Services that would give your child full Medicaid which translates to coverage for speech, occupational, physical, and behavioral therapies, as well as dia-

pers, and potty training, respite care and even more. It is not based on your income. The child, who has no income, calculates it. You must first be a client of Developmental Services to qualify. This is an arduous process, and they usually have long waiting lists. Get signed up as soon as your child is diagnosed, no matter where he/she is on the spectrum. This will be a big help down the road. It is better to have it available and not need it, than to not be able to receive it.

> We celebrate the fact that he is quirky and interesting and doesn't always care whether people understand or accept him because he isn't a social butterfly. This builds his character for the future when others say it can't be done. Alex will say, "Oh yes it can, let me show you how!"
>
> Debbie (mom)

10. *Be patient.* Patience, patience, and more patience. This is what you will need on a daily basis. As I stated before, sometimes you just need to pull yourself aside and take a breather. I remember several times trying to get Charlie in the bathtub. It would be a 45–60 minute screaming and hitting match because he did not want to get in it. Sometimes I would succumb and say "fine" because I could not physically get him in the tub by myself. Other times, by the time I got him in it, I was soaked as well. Once he got in the tub and it was the same process getting him out. Sometimes his baths could take a total of almost three hours...talk about a much-needed breather after we are done with those. He also struggles with keeping his emotions on an even keel.

He will be fine one minute and then just start crying out of the blue. As soon as you start worrying about him he is fine. It really messes with your emotions as well. Just know they are just like you and me, but they are unable to convey their true feelings and sometimes they just come tumbling out. All we can do is be patient and be there for them to lean on.

> Having a child with asperger's is an absolute blessing. It is not always easy, but it is definitely a gift.
>
> Cori (parent)

11. *Find good support.* This is so important. Find a friend, family member, buddy from church, or anyone you can feel free to talk to who will listen. They don't need to understand everything; they just need to listen to you. Getting your feelings and frustrations out is key. The worst thing you can do is keep all this in.

Autism will affect all areas of your life. Sometimes marriages are tested when you travel this journey. My husband and I became even closer than we already were. We helped each other with our different struggles we were having. Everyone handles stress differently, so try and find someone that you can air out your thoughts with and feel comfortable with to share what is going on with you. This was pretty hard for me to do. I will have to admit. I am the type of person who doesn't want to burden anyone, but I know now that this is key if you really want to help your child with autism. If you are falling apart, you can't do the best for your child. Remember you have to take care of the people who are trying to help your child...and that is *you.*

> We get the greatest joy out of simple accomplishments he achieves. That is what this is all about; helping the kids reach goals. Seeing the smallest of gains I see in my son makes me feel happy and blessed everyday.
>
> Wendy (mom)

12. *Start Applied Behavior Analysis.* This treatment is the only scientific proven method that improves human behavior. When someone can't communicate effectively they may engage in inappropriate behavior. Applied Behavior Analysis is a behavioral approach that uses reinforcement as the primary treatment. It can change lives, not just kids with autism but anyone that uses this method. (I have even used this on my husband.)

The focus is on increasing compliance, not punishing non-compliance. I was really bad about saying over and over what Charlie did wrong instead of focusing and reinforcing what he did correct and also reinforcing new appropriate behavior. You want to replace inappropriate behavior with appropriate behavior by reinforcement. Behavior Analysts pick socially significant behaviors and choose an intervention that will help bring changes to improve a person's life. It is only covered by insurance in a few states (South Carolina, Texas, and Pennsylvania). Other states are working on getting insurance mandated for ABA services. The therapy can be either one hour a week or more than 40 hours per week. Each child is different and a behavioral assessment would need to be completed to know how many hours behavior analysis is needed. One critical piece of advice about this is to be careful. There are some "clinicians" out there calling themselves "behaviorists, behavior analysts, or behavior specialists" that are not board certified in behavior analysis. If this method is "being taught" by someone who is not board certified it could lead to more problem behaviors. It has to be done by someone who has been trained in behavior analysis and who has been certified. You can go on the behavior analyst's website and lookup the clinician's license to check if they are a legitimate behavior analyst: www.bacb.com.

> We decided long ago to take it a day at a time and not to worry about his failures, but to praise him for his goals and accomplishments. He is our gift from God, our handsome boy, Flavio.
>
> Matha (mother)

13. *Be positive.* I know that some days I wonder where I can reach for strength, but I always seem to find it. When I first started putting this book together, I asked a large amount of people to share their stories with me so I could pass them along to you. I would ask them how autism has been a blessing to them. Probably more than 50 percent of the people I questioned told me outright that there are no blessings with autism. I purposely asked some people repeatedly, because I wanted them to be forced to think of the positive things that have happened to them since autism had come into their lives.

When I look at the positive aspects of autism, it helps me see what my purpose here on earth is. Yes it is hard, yes it is trying, yes it is exhausting at times, but I have seen many more positives that have come out of this than negative. You can have ten great things happen to you today and then only one negative thing, and sometimes that one negative thing can cloud all those ten great things. Try to focus on the positive including what your child can do and what your child has shown you about life and love.

> Zackery is a great, big brother to his two year old sister and he is one of the most loving people I have ever met. Zackery has taught me to appreciate the little accomplishments in life that most parents overlook. Patience and understanding have taken on a new meaning in our household, thanks to him.
>
> Esmeralda (mother)

> We need to teach others in our society to appreciate the many gifts (especially of the heart) of autistic children. My children challenge and teach me new things everyday. We appreciate every thing they learn and take nothing for granted. I also have been able to give hope to and console other mothers of autistic children, and this has been rewarding.
>
> Michele (mother)

> My son was diagnosed approximately five years ago with high functioning (SM) autism. He didn't speak for almost eight years of his life, with the exception of his family inside his home. He has started therapies, medication, and numerous other treatments and has been a real joy to our family!

Julie (mother)

God in his infinite wisdom gave me exactly what I needed, regardless of what I thought I wanted. Matthew builds me up every day and fills my heart with joy. Together, we appreciate each day and the little triumphs that take on so much more meaning when autism enters the picture. True, we are still working on the "easy going" part, and our journey is far from over. But we need to have something to keep working towards, now don't we?

Emily (mother)

These kids hear what we say about them. They are extremely smart. Don't discourage them by making them believe that they have to fit into some scientific mold that society has placed on them. Instead encourage them and allow them to see that you believe in them and their abilities to do anything they set out to do. This will make your life, and more importantly your children's life, have worth. In our opinion God doesn't make mistakes, Zackery was made just the way God intended him to be.

Esmeralda (mother)

We are blessed with a very loving child. He is only three and a half years old, diagnosed with autism only a year ago, so we do not know if he'll ever learn to talk or write. All we know is that he is one of the happiest children we have ever met and we are blessed to be chosen by God to be his parents. And our responsibility as his parents is the make sure we do everything in our power to do everything possible to make sure that he is the man that God has intended him to be.

Megan (mother)

My son is two and he is a blessing all by himself. He finally hugs me and that is something that I longed for. We have a busy day now with teachers and therapies but we get through it. God gave me this child and I intend to help him live his life to the fullest. I was born to be his mommy and he was born to be my child, I couldn't ask for more.

Jennifer (mother)

Over the course of time he has grown into a smart young man. I put him in a very small private school where he is flourishing, and the outburst, which were always the problem, have since ceased. I believe Zak will do just fine in the world, and I have no doubts about his future. I now know two other parents with kids (boys) who come to me for advice about their kids, and I now can help them understand them better.

Sherri (mom)

WHAT ABOUT SCHOOL?

Consider it all joy, my brethren, when you encounter various trials, knowing that the testing of your faith produces endurance. And let endurance have its perfect result, that you may be perfect and complete, lacking in nothing.
James 1:2–4 (NAS)

Choosing a school is probably one of the most important things you will do for your child. Once you have registered them and gotten their evaluations completed with the school system, you will be scheduled to meet for an IEP meeting. This is a journey that you will be on until they are out of school. IEP stands for Individual Educational Plan. This program is through your local school system. If your child is under three, he or she is eligible for early intervention assistance. This is a federally funded program called Part C. If your child is older than three, you need to call Developmental Services and the Exceptional Education Department. Your child is guaranteed a free, appropriate, public education from age three to twenty-one. This is supplied by your local school district.

> My mother told me that you are a part of a special club to get one of these kids...fun kids who have an interesting perspective on what life has to offer. The scary part is that these kids don't have a disability...they have a learning difference...they are socially linear and are a product of the environment. They don't enjoy beating around the bush and point out to us as grownups that we make things too complicated. They show us the simpler ways to do things and remind us that boundaries are something that we impose, to maintain control and safety. Eating is not a big deal and sleeping is optional. Getting creative to communicate is absolutely essential and requires us to use a different part of our brain.
>
> Damarius (mom)

Our journey began when we learned of the FDLRS (Florida Diagnostic and Learning Resources System) program. This program, for ages 0–3, is called Child Find. Charlie had just turned three. We called the diagnostic center early July 2004 to get an appointment for an evaluation for services. The first available appointment was for the middle of August, so I quickly grabbed it. My husband took Charlie by himself since I had to run our business. I was the only one who could run the office.

The evaluation took place at an elementary school full of long lines of kids and parents waiting to be evaluated. Charlie did not like it at all. He was scared and was screaming and crying. He did not like big crowds or loud places. The lady that was scheduling all the evaluations noticed

Charlie having a hard time. My husband quickly filled out all the forms, and she took them right in. My husband explained that our son had recently turned three and was diagnosed with autism spectrum disorder. She attempted to do a hearing test, but could not do it with him. He did not understand what she was asking, and could not answer if he was or wasn't hearing a certain tone. She called his name when he was turned around, and he turned and looked at her. She signed off on a paper that said he was eligible for services. The next step was to be evaluated by a psychologist, as well as speech and occupational therapists. Within the school system, this process took about three months. Once the evaluations were complete, we made an appointment to sit down with the evaluators and discuss the results.

I remember the day very clearly. I was a little anxious as to what they would say. I still had this little bit of hope that they would say he is fine, and he just needs to do this, this, and this. I was praying for a great report and still thinking that all the doctors had gotten it all wrong somehow. Tony and I brought Charlie to the school where they requested the meeting. Hardly anyone was at the school. We met with a school psychologist, speech and language pathologist, school director, and the school board representative. The school board representative started the meeting by explaining how we would discuss Charlie. They would go around the table, each giving their findings. The psychologist gave each of us a copy of her seven-page evaluation. Charlie had never been this thoroughly evaluated, or been seen by a psychologist.

> My brother struggles understanding many things, yet he seems to understand the concept of perfect love better than anyone I have ever

> met. I was about six years old when I remember Zach being diagnosed. I remember him being extremely irritable even for a baby, and how he would zone out for hours at a time. I remember seeing my parents nearly at the breaking point of frustration, and not being able to help.
>
> Seth (brother)

The psychologist explained the various tests she had completed and her results in detail. She basically read the whole evaluation aloud and would stop at times to explain her comments a little further if needed. She started with all the statistics like his age, reason for testing, etc. They conducted these tests in late September when he was a little over three years of age. Her report went on to explain what our concerns were and what difficulties he was having. For instance, it stated, "Sometimes he likes to be left alone and is easily upset. He has difficulty sitting still, acts impulsively, and spends less than five minutes on most activities. He has difficulty making changes in his routine or activities."

Then the report described her behavioral observations and impressions, "He used toys functionally but also lined up the cars or grouped them together and liked spinning the blades on the helicopter. He became frightened of a toy when it began making high-pitched noises. Charles also became agitated when the examiners spoke to him too loudly and when a toy cellular phone went off. He would make fleeting eye contact."

Next came the difficult part. Up until that point I knew and observed on a daily basis everything on the reports. The next sentence was tough to hear. "In terms of cognitive or pre-academic functioning, Charles' skills are demonstrated at the 26-month level of development." I remember thinking, *okay, that is only a year behind. We can deal with this.* Then she talked about independent functioning. "Charles' self-help skills are demonstrated at the 20-month level of development." I again thought, *okay this is a little worse, but we can help him get through this.* Social/behavioral was the next section we needed to go over. The psychologist explained all the various tests she performed such as the Childhood Autism Rating Scale (CARS) and the Autism Behavior Checklist (ABC). On the CARS test, his score was 40, which put him in the severely autistic range. The ABC test revealed he was in the average range.

> The innocence that these children possess is hard to describe. The beauty they see, we tend to overlook. When I go with my two little ones to the store the first thing that they want to do is go to the flower section and smell the flowers. I have never once seen other parents with their children doing that. My children are extremely happy children, they look forward to every day. They wake up and go to bed with smiles on their faces.
>
> Gabi (mother)

The psychologist generally talked about his results and then stated, "These results indicate that Charles displays many of the behavioral characteristics commonly associated with autism spectrum disorder." Wow! I felt that knife again go in my chest. My hopes dashed again. I thought to myself, here is another professional saying that he has autism. I wanted to run from that room and burst into tears, but I knew I had to sit there and listen to three more pages of evaluation. I had a hard time breathing and my heart was racing very fast. The room was spinning and everything they said now was like an echo. I was saying lots of prayers to myself like, *Lord, please help me to hear these words they are saying about my son.*

Next on the evaluation was the topic of communication. The psychologist said, "Charles presents with a severe delay in his pragmatic, receptive, and expressive language skills. He communicates primarily through gestures, jargon, gibberish, and limited, one-word utterances to get his needs met. Receptive language skills were demonstrated at the nine-month level of development. Expressive language skills were demonstrated at the nine-month level of development." I couldn't even look up. My eyes were full of tears by then. Tony was sitting next to me, but I could not even look at him. I kept hearing "he is at a nine-month-old level." It rang over and over in my head.

How can this be? What did I do to my son? I went back to that first day he was diagnosed. Did I eat something wrong to make him like this? Did I not get enough sleep when I was pregnant? Did my grief over my uncle's death make him this way? Did I not eat enough vegetables? What did I do wrong?

She finished the report with a summary of why she felt he was eligible for the autism program. I just started to cry at this point and felt such horrible grief. Remarkably, they were all so supportive. They kept reassuring me that if we continue to get him these services and therapies, he would be just fine.

> My beautiful daughter was diagnosed with PDD-NOS at age three, she is now six and has overcome most of her challenges, and very

> much a typical child. It has been a blessing in so many ways in my life...a few of the biggest ones were realizing that there is so much more to life than having a stressful, high- paying job, and all of the luxuries that go with it. A year after her diagnosis, my husband and I made a very difficult decision, I left my high- paying, corporate job to be with my daughter and get her as much intervention as possible, and it has paid off two fold.
>
> Kimberley (mom)

The next step was for the team to let me know their school placement recommendations. They had one opening left at Nova (Bauduin School) in Davie, Florida. I was so happy. My husband was not from this area, so he had no idea what great news that was. They have a full autistic program. It is the best of the best. Some families move to this area just so their child can attend this school.

He went for the first time during the last week of October. I remember all of us walking in as a family, Tony, me, Chelsea, and of course Charlie. It looked like a mansion. It was gorgeous. The people there were so great and helpful. The most important thing was that they liked Charlie. He had such excellent teachers and aides. Ms. Sirlon was a god-send. She really helped Charlie so much. He also had Ms. Stephanie and Ms. Jenna of whom he loved as well. They were very important to our family and gave us lots of hope on this journey that we were on.

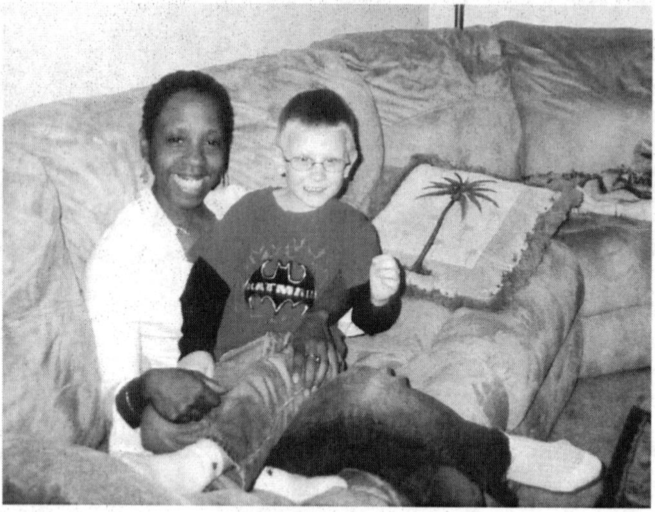

Ms. Sirlon, his teacher/therapist, at Bauduin School, Oct. 2004.

During this time our family made some major life decisions. We decided back in May (before Charlie was diagnosed) that we needed to make some changes for our family. We were not happy living in Fort Lauderdale. I felt it wasn't the best choice to raise my family. We had always talked about moving to Central Florida, but thought it would never be possible because of our business, All Southern Care Rehabilitation.

In May of 2004, we decided to buy a house in a beautiful new community called Lakes of Windermere. Our original decision was to buy while the prices were low enough and eventually later move the family there. Once we put some money down on the house, we really started to think more and more about our business. We provided therapists for home-health agencies and saw patients for them. Because we ran it out of our garage, I was able to be with the kids and watch them while I worked.

> A lot of parents do not even realize how precious it is to have a child reach a milestone, no matter how small. Not only do I realize it, but I treasure each and every one and celebrate like he won the Super Bowl.
>
> Estelle (mother)

Tony and I talked first about dwindling the company down gradually. Then he would find a therapy job up in the Orlando/Windermere area. Tony had earned his physical therapist assistant license in 2001. Then all of a sudden I realized how much work we had put into making the business successful for almost 10 years. Perhaps someone would pay us to take it over. I had already done all the hard work; they would just have to keep it going and maybe even develop it a little further. Even though it was hard to turn down business, I had purposely kept it fairly small so that I could take care of my family and do the job well. I would rather keep a small number of agencies happy and do a great job than keep a few happy and do a fair job.

We called a business broker in late May. He gave us a figure of what the company would be worth, and we started the process of trying to find a buyer. We told *no one* of what we were doing, because we had no idea how long the process would take. Little did we know it would only take about six months. Needless to say, it became a stressful time. I was trying to run the business, trying to sell the business, pack, get Charlie to his various therapy sessions, trying to keep the plan for the business quiet and still trying to understand autism. We had three hurricanes come through our area all at this same time. Besides Tony's cancer and my dad's death, this had become the most difficult time of my life. It was very scary in all directions. With all my praying, God was definitely saying, "oh it is Patty again!"

> Many times I feel she is not listening or paying attention, but again she lets me know she is listening. Several years ago in Church the Priest was talking about the Holy Spirit in the form of a Dove. I was holding Christy and she picked up her head and loudly said "that is 105 on your radio dial!" She is a sweet little girl who charms so many people, her teachers love her and always comment that they feel she is a special child and are glad to have had her. She is truly my blessing from God.
>
> Linda (adoptive mother)

Once we had a confirmed bid on our business, we really decided to move our family to Windermere. Construction of the house would not be complete for a few more months. Out of nowhere, two guys, Gary and Lawrence, from New York, decided to buy our business! We closed on our business on November 4, 2004. I was just as nervous as I had been on my wedding day. Overall though, I was happy to let it go, because I needed all my time now to concentrate on Charlie and Chelsea. As a part of our contract, we agreed to help train them until December 22. We were trying to pack our house, get the kids registered for different schools in Windermere, train these guys to run the company, and help Charlie with all his therapies and school. On top of all of this I fractured one of my toes and was hobbling around. It was overwhelming. There were so many unknowns. What would happen to Charlie? What school would he go to? Where would Tony work? We eventually figured out all these answers soon enough.

It all came together. We were fully moved to Windermere by the end of January. We had a meeting with the Orange County school system on the following Wednesday. We gave them copies of all of Charlie's old IEP's (Individual Education Plan) so they would know all the services Broward County was giving him. In Broward, he had a full- time speech therapy teacher and he was just approved for occupational therapy once a week and the summer ESY (Extended School Year) program. Tony gave the paperwork to the school but they wanted to do new evaluations for speech therapy and occupational therapy. We also learned that they didn't have a private day school like what he had in Fort Lauderdale. The program they offered was only two and a half hours however, and it was all they offered. At the school in Ft. Lauderdale he went from 8:00 a.m. until 2:30 everyday, Monday through Friday. We were not happy so far with what they were telling us. By the time they have snack, go to the bathroom, and go on the playground, what were they going to teach my son? A two and a half hour program I would call daycare, not teaching. The worst part was he was not getting therapy. We decided to enroll him so that he would be getting something until I could find something better. We kept asking about his therapy and they would say, "We will check on it."

> What a blessing that autism has become! At first I had responded much like most father's would, I was angry as well as disappointed. I felt

> that God had taken my little boy's ability to live life at it's fullest, and replaced it with constant, utter chaos with no chance to accomplish any of (my) goals and dreams for him. I was selfish and wanted the ultimate athlete, a son that I could be proud of! Charlie has a mother that cares so deeply for him that she puts her own physical well being to the side to attend to his emotional well being. I am so proud of her because, despite her own short comings (in her mind) she is one of the strongest individuals I have ever met, and I truly do thank God everyday that he put her into my life.
>
> Tony (father)

In the midst of all of this, Tony's dad died at Duke Hospital in North Carolina on March 1, 2005. Tony was gone for 10 days. It was so difficult for both of us but more for him. I needed his support so much especially with Charlie, but I wanted to be there for him with his father's loss. While he was gone, I found a school about 10 minutes from our house called United Cerebral Palsy Preschool. It was a charter school. The school system would pay for it, but I would have to drive him because they said they don't provide busing. We enrolled him in the Orange County school system February 2, 2005, and they didn't evaluate him for speech until March 15th and occupational therapy until March 22nd. It took them a month and a half to two months to do those evaluations. In the meantime he had not received any therapy for over two months. We had decided to transfer him to UCP the last week of March. He did really well there. His teachers, Ms. Melinda, and Ms. Norma were great with him.

We met again with the school district for another IEP. Since Charlie left Bauduin in the middle of January until April 18, he had not received any speech or occupational therapy treatments. That is a total of *three months* that he never got any therapy. I tried my best to work with him but I am not a "professional." I was unhappy, needless to say. The meeting did not go very well. They had a speech therapist, occupational therapist, and a school board representative there. Tony and I sat listening to some of them tell lie after lie and I called them on every one.

The speech therapist was very, very nice and she again recommended speech therapy three times a week (30 minute sessions) just like what he was receiving in Ft. Lauderdale. The occupational therapist was defensive from the first word she spoke. She went on to explain in her own way that Charlie did not need occupational therapy. She said he could manipulate the scissors by himself. However, when my husband pressed her on it she admitted that he needed maximum assistance. Her evaluation report said, "Based on the results of this evaluation and the guidelines of the CERT, educationally relevant occupational therapy may not be indicated at this time." She also admitted that she evaluated him four times and combined the fourth evaluation with another boy's. Most therapists only need to see a child one time to do their initial evaluation and give their recommendations. Why was she proud that it took her four sessions to figure out what his needs were? While she was so proud of how long it took, my son was not getting his therapy that the school district legally agreed upon in the previous November, for which this school district was very aware of. Then she was proud to tell us she saw my son and another boy in the same classroom and did the evaluations simultaneously. This is clearly against the Florida Board of Occupational Therapy. You cannot conduct an evaluation on someone and be watching another child at the same time.

The occupational therapist should be focused only on one child when he/she is performing the evaluation.

> When the ultrasound revealed that my first born would be male…I told myself I don't know anything about raising boys. I prayed every day that our son would be healthy, happy, and easygoing, with plenty of friends and smart, sweet, loving and kind. I felt much more prepared to raise girls, but I believed that by getting the "perfect" boy, I would stand a chance at being a successful mother to him.
>
> Emily (mother)

We kept asking why his ST (speech therapy) and OT (occupational therapy) were not just being transferred. Why did we have to start all over again? And why are they telling me that he doesn't even need OT? None of this made sense to me. How are they going to fix this? They said they weren't able to change the form that sat in front of us, but yet they were using white correction tape all over it for other errors they had made. That made no sense to me. I was informed before the meeting that if I didn't feel comfortable with what they were offering, I shouldn't sign the papers, but ask for copies to look over for a few days. Well, as soon as I informed them that I wouldn't be signing that day and would take a few days to look over the forms both the OT and the County Coordinator threatened me. They warned that if I didn't immediately sign those forms that Charlie wouldn't get his ST, and we wouldn't be back to meet for another month. They got loud with their voices and both their bodies moved closer to me across the table. Why were they so defensive and anxious for me to sign those papers right away? I started to laugh out of surprise at how afraid they were I wouldn't sign them.

Against our better judgment, Tony and I did sign their papers. All Individual Education Plans have a time frame of how long you have to change the plan. Be aware of this. Just because you sign the IEP, it doesn't mean you still can't change something on it. Speech therapy was the most important thing for Charlie to be receiving, so we didn't want any more delay with that issue. I found out later that it states that even if we didn't sign the IEP they were responsible to start the speech therapy services since it was on the IEP. We set up another meeting to discuss further OT. We all agreed to forget the first OT evaluation that was done in March that stated he did not need OT. The occupational therapist would look into why Charlie didn't get the OT in the transfer. Interestingly enough my husband got a call from the OT a couple days later. They had decided to give him the OT that he had missed once a week, and also give him the visits he had missed for almost three months.

We sat down again with them the first week of May 2005 and signed a new IEP that gave him OT one time a week and ST three times a week until the next annual review, which was the first week in April 2006. We were finally okay, but why did this have to take over three months and about four meetings? What a mess! Needless to say, I was exhausted from dealing with this mess. I was in a new town and trying to help with the transitions for the kids. It was a tough time for all of us.

The next IEP meeting was at the end of March 2006, and it was for our annual review of Charlie's services. Just prior to the meeting, actually in the same week, I received notes in Charlie's box that both his occupational therapist and his speech therapist that worked at UCP were quitting. There was no notice. I was patient. I understood things happen, but I felt the charter school (UCP) would still provide somehow, or make up for any sessions he would miss since they are receiving governmental funds to provide these services. A couple weeks passed and I realized he still was not receiving ST or OT. I asked the school director about it. His response was that he was getting an occupational therapist from another center to help out until they found another and they found a speech therapist but were just waiting for all her paperwork/background check to come back. Finally he got services and I spoke to both therapists prior to the annual IEP meeting. I also found out he had missed five OT and six ST sessions during this transition, so I mentioned it in the IEP meeting and asked how we could get those made up. The school director quickly brushed us off and told us he would talk to us later about it. I questioned the director at a later time about when Charlie would be getting those OT and ST visits made up that they did not have staff for. He told me that it is out of his control when he loses staff and that "the kids that really needed the therapy were seen." So Charlie, in his mind, didn't really need ST and OT. I can't believe a director of a school would make a comment like that to a parent. I know when we owned our own therapy company, I had therapists quit, get sick or maybe have a death in the family and patients still needed to be seen. Life just doesn't stop and care doesn't cease just because you have employees quit. I would have never told a patients family, *well we covered the patients that really needed treatment but for you we won't be able to make up the last two weeks they weren't given therapy.* I was fuming after our conversation, to say the least. The IEP meeting went smoothly and his teacher, the OT representative, and the ST representative were all there to review therapy goals and treatment plans before the county coordinator. Everyone agreed that Charlie would continue ST three times a week and OT once a week. We all signed the paper and were set for smooth sailing...or so we thought.

> On the verge of delivering our second child, I attempted to console our unreachable child after being awoken almost every night by Matthew's ear-shattering screams. These screams would continue as long episodes during which we could do nothing to calm him. The intensity of these episodes was unlike anything we had experienced before, and sitting helplessly on the sidelines while Matthew suffered through them, was both heartbreaking and terrifying.
>
> Emily (mother)

A couple of weeks later, on a Monday, I dropped off Charlie at school at 8:30 a.m. and was given a small note that read: "Mrs. Myers, go and see Orange County schools at 8:30am Monday." I asked his teacher what this was about and she had no idea. I walked around the corner to the office, and the coordinator looked very happy to see me. I sat down and she blurted out, "We made a mistake. Charlie should not have received OT. We need you to sign consent for a new evaluation. He was only given OT last time because that is what came from Broward. He needs a new evaluation to see if he really needs this anymore." I was sure and told her that I knew they wanted a new evaluation in order to stop his OT. If the goals and treatment were not appropriate, why did Orange County sit and listen to the OT and agree to continue with these new goals and treatments? I told her that I needed to talk with my husband first.

The following Thursday in the mail we received another notice for a meeting for the following Monday morning to get consent for OT/PT evaluations. My husband called the school director to say we would not be attending the meeting because we had decided to first seek legal counsel regarding the matter. Nothing was said to me Monday when I dropped/picked Charlie up. Tuesday was Charlie's regular OT day, and when I dropped him off, the occupational therapist told me she had been informed that Charlie would no longer be receiving OT. She gave me some copies of specific things to work on with him. I quickly corrected her and alerted her that it was still being discussed. After getting in the car, I realized she told me Charlie wouldn't be receiving OT. When I went to pick Charlie up from school later that day, the receptionist informed me effective today he would not be receiving anymore OT. I was livid. How can they just stop services? I have a legal document that they need to follow. I decided to contact further legal counsel and got help right away with the Advocacy Center for Disabilities.

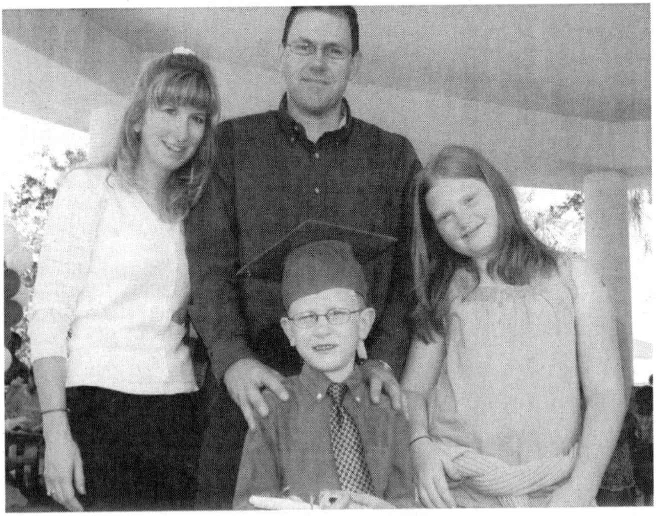

Charlie graduates from UCP Pre-School May 2006

We then met again to sit down with his teachers from his new school, Thornebrooke Elementary. Charlie was going to start Kindergarten. I was so excited. I requested another IEP in order to transfer him to this new school. I assumed that since the district stopped his OT without informing us in May, that no OT services would show up on his IEP. Well much to our surprise he was given OT again on this IEP. At first, nothing was mentioned of it. The county was just going to act like the situation never occurred. We requested a physical therapy evaluation because, for a couple of years, one of his toes has been crossing over another one. Without correction, this could become a real balance problem for him. He also uses both shoulders to cover his ears a lot and we are concerned about his posture if he keeps it up. When the district personnel handed us a consent form to sign for PT in order for an evaluation to be made, they tried to have us sign a consent also at the same time for ST and

OT. The nightmare was starting all over again. They cannot evaluate your child without your written consent. We had already been given approval for ST and OT visits and now the district was wanting us to let them evaluate Charlie all over again for ST and OT so the district could then turn around and try and deny him services.

> I love him like no other and when we go to the park and he just swings for hours and doesn't pay attention to anything but the swing. I never feel bad because the other kids are playing and laughing as they run around the playground, instead I hold my head up high knowing God has given me a chance to be a mother and love this little boy no matter who he is or how he is and that is all I wanted out of life; to love a child and be a mother.
>
> Jennifer (mom)

I asked the county representative why she stopped services without our consent and her comment was, "I am not at liberty to discuss it."

The advocacy center was on conference call hearing all this. She spoke up and said, "You are not at liberty to discuss this child? I don't understand. You can take away services without any regard to letting the parents be aware, but you can't talk about it?" The advocate asked how we could rectify this situation because the head of the district, wanted it all to be rectified during the meeting.

The representative recommended that she draft a letter to the district of our concerns. This was done and the district agreed to give Charlie the missed OT visits and to continue his OT one time a week as the IEP stated he should have. Thanks to the help from the Advocacy Center and Selina this was made possible. It is really tough to have so many meetings about things that the district is supposed to be doing. We as families are already so busy enough helping our children and all these meetings and studying about the law really takes away from us spending time with our kids.

For his first year in Kindergarten, we were very pleased with his new school. It is a public school, but they have an autism program and have an inclusion program as well. An inclusion program is where they have the children with autism in the same population as the regular education children for different periods of time. This might mean just one class, or they might be in a regular education class the entire time with the help of an aide. There are three teachers and only eight children in the autism resource class he was in. They have lots of PECS (Picture Exchange Communication System), which has really helped my son. He is such a visual learner.

> I am a single parent with two autistic children, six and four years old. I think I am blessed. I don't think parents really appreciate what God has given to them until they have children that have special needs. I would never change my children for "typical" children. They have taught me patience and unconditional love. Every simple goal they reach is like climbing a mountain.
>
> Gabi (mother)

At the end of his first year of Kindergarten, his teachers

recommended that he should stay back in kindergarten for the next year as well. Charlie hadn't quite mastered all of the kindergarten requirements. He was only 5 at the end of this year because he has a July birthday. He was the youngest in his class. At our IEP meeting in March, we had also discussed putting him in a regular education class one to two hours a day with the help of an aide. Our plan was to slowly transition him in the regular education class and mainstream him.

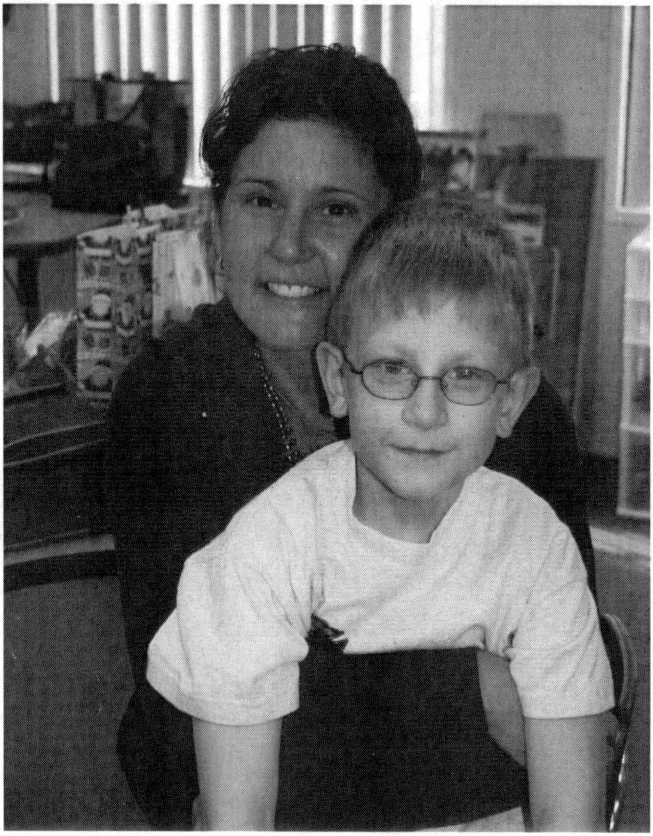

Ms. Kim, Special Ed teacher (Thornebrooke Elementary) and Charlie December 2007

We started the second year of kindergarten a little rocky from the start. From the first day he was put in the regular education class almost 80 percent of the day, and then was transitioned into the autism resource room the rest of the day. I was pretty nervous considering he had never been in a regular education classroom, never been in a classroom with more than 12 children and less than three to four teachers/ paraprofessionals. This regular education classroom had 19 children and *one* teacher. I had a little anxiety to say the least. The first week of school was horrible. He could not tell us "how school was." He could not say if he liked it or not. He could not say if it was hard. He could not tell us what he even did that day. His behaviors were increasing in severity. By the third night, my husband and I just lay in the bed and cried. He was screaming, laughing, singing, hitting himself, and laying on the floor with his eyes closed and rambling sentences that made no sense to us at all. Charlie was on overload. He held it together so well all day long and then when he would get home, would totally break down. It broke our hearts. Seeing him this way only made my anxiety worse. What is going on at school? Is he doing okay? Is someone telling him to go to the bathroom? Is someone making fun of him?

About a month into school I decided I would visit both of his classrooms all day to see what was happening. I also wanted to see how I could implement anything that they are doing to help him at home. I had gotten several reports saying that he was "doing great," "fits right in," and "he's doing fine." It was a tough day for me. At first I noticed in the general education classroom that he was quiet, he whispered, he sat in his seat nicely etc. On the outside he did look "great," he did look "fine." He had trouble with the reading lab, he did not like to put on the head phones. The class was directed to be on page two and he was on page six (he had already completed pages two-five). He was at a fine motor rotation with another little boy. This is an activity that helps kids work with and manipulate small things with their hands. The boy was teasing and making fun of how Charlie would roll his eyes and chew on his tongue. Charlie was starring off into space during "big group reading time." When he was in the small reading group he had his head laying on his arm, which was on the desk. The teacher would ask the class questions and the class would raise their hands and the teacher would call on them. I never saw Charlie raise his hand. I don't think he understood some of the questions anyway.

I looked at my watch, and it was 1:00, no one had ever told him to go to the bathroom. We were *still* potty training him. Yes, he was six years old. He only wears pull-ups at night but we are still trying to get him to initiate going on his own. If you don't tell him to go every hour or so then he will just go in his pants and he doesn't even care. I had explained this to both teachers at the beginning of the year. At the end of that day, I was discouraged because I felt that my son was not getting the kind of immediate reinforcement that he needs to achieve in his academics. But his social and communication skills were doing great, I could see vast improvements in those areas.

We had another IEP meeting in October to go over these issues that I saw in his general education setting and to ask why his IEP was not being followed . We hired an attorney (Danny). He was and is a great support. Orange County brought their attorney as well. It was a meeting that lasted four hours and was still not completed. The county decided they needed data on Charlie being in the regular education classroom to see if he really needed a supportive aide. Their attorney stated, "I just don't see the need for supportive aides at this time." We also reviewed how non-compliant they had been with his IEP.

We decided to go back to the original IEP that stated he be in regular education only one to two hours a day. They took data and it clearly showed that he needed the help of a supportive aide. It showed how he got frustrated easily and needed more reinforcement and help in certain areas. We didn't want an aide to be with him every single minute, but we saw how easily he could slip through the cracks. Charlie had difficulty with transitioning certain times of the day. I was frustrated that we had to waste another month collecting data when they should have done this from the beginning of the year. Why do we as parents have to request everything? My nerves were pretty shot at this point.

We met again for another IEP meeting in December. Tony and I prayed before the meeting and asked God to give us wisdom, a clear mind, and peace. We had brought our attorney again and also a court reporter. Yes, you heard me...a court reporter. I decided to bring a court reporter because the district kept saying, "Ms. Myers, I think you misunderstood me, or Ms. Myers, that is not what I said." I wanted to make sure that everything was documented so there would be no issue on what was actually said. It worked out wonderfully. Orange County also brought their attorney. They were not too happy with the sight of the court reporter. I had prior to the meeting noted that we would be bringing a court reporter. Sometimes you have to do whatever it takes to get the services you know your child *requires* to be successful, and you know the federal government has made available. This is what FAPE is for...free and appropriate education. It is unfortunate that *free* education turns into you paying for an attorney and a court reporter.

The Orange County attorney was late a half hour to both IEP meetings. I am sure that wasn't accidental. It didn't hurt us at all, we could stay for hours, but it was very rude and inconsiderate. I am sure if we showed up a half hour late they would have started the meeting without us. The meeting concluded with what we had been asking for since day one. Charlie would be in full inclusion with the help of a supportive aide at certain times of his academics. He would not have an aide walking around with him, but she would be used during reading and academic times where he needs some reinforcement. He will be in the regular education class all day long. It is crazy that we have to have all these meetings, pay an attorney, pay a court reporter, have 10 to 12 people discussing the same issues over and over, collect data just to come to the original conclusion that we as parents requested from the beginning. The point in telling our history is to show that you *must not give up*. They will *try* to intimidate you, they will tell you *no*, they will try and strong arm you, but you have to stay strong. You need to educate yourself. You need to have a good support system, and most importantly, you have to do what is appropriate for your child and continue to-request the services that they need.

> In my travels, God has also put many non-believers in my life, they all wondered how I stayed so calm and did so much. I was able to share with them my views and beliefs, and my positive attitude and beliefs have made a difference in their life along with coping with their child's disability. My daughter is exactly the person that God intended her to be, she is fulfilling God's purpose for her, and she is the biggest blessing in my life and many others.
>
> Kimberley (mother)

Some school districts only get a slap on the wrist for not following the law. They know there is no real consequence so they basically do what they want to. If you are having difficulty, my advice is to get in touch with your state leaders, including your senators and representatives, and let them know the problems or concerns you have with your school district.

Parents should step up and realize that they can change laws and make the school leaders accountable to make the right decisions for these children. Unfortunately, parents hardly have time for this after we have spent most of our time each day just trying to help our kids. I have found that email is the best way to communicate to our leaders. It is quick, easy, and creates a paper trail. Someone once told me in the midst of all our difficulties getting Charlie his services that, "Only the squeaky wheel gets oiled." They also said, "You are not here to make friends, you are just here to get Charlie what he requires." It is a business meeting, it is not personal. I have repeated both of those statements to myself, especially in our IEP meetings. I also think that we need to praise our teachers, paraprofessionals, lunch personnel, crossing guards, bus drivers, administration, and anyone else who is involved in your child's education that has done a good job. It is easy to say what is wrong, but remember to point out what has been working as well.

It is always a struggle to get the services that your child needs. The school district doesn't look at your child as a person that needs help. They usually see them as a cost factor. They have a form called "the Matrix." It asks questions about your child, and based on his needs, he is given a number. That number correlates with how much money the state will pay for your child for that particular school year. Autism is generally one of the highest numbers calculated.

That is one reason why the school district tried to take away Charlie's OT.

> Do miracles happen? Without a doubt. My son just saw the neurologist for Madison and she no longer displayed autistic behavior. He said he "had" to remove the label. Please, all parents, all family, all grandparents, join me in hoping and praying, do not accept the negative comments, the articles that try to "doom" us to something they do not even understand. All things are possible. I raise a glass to miracles waiting to happen!
>
> Janice from Brooklyn (grandma)

The budget seems to be the school districts main concern. You will hear how they made this decision on what is best for the child, but that is hardly ever true. The really sad part, I think, is that if the school district took the time and energy to help these kids in the earlier years, they wouldn't be paying for as much care when they became adults. My advice is to stay strong. When you have an IEP meeting, treat it as a sales meeting. Don't get emotional, and stick to your guns. Take a friend with you if you need to for support. I sat in on an IEP meeting with my friend and even asked a few questions for her and the school seemed to be worried about who I was. The school staff and district staff will try to intimidate you, but stand your ground, because they won't be there for you when your child is 22 and is not able to take care of himself. I can't say it enough, educate yourself on the law.

I also recommend that you research anything they tell

you. Make sure that it is the truth. Often, they stretch the truth to benefit their budget or lack of available staff. I decided finally to join them instead of fight with them. I am now on my son's Autism Committee PTA and am trying to be a part of the team instead of their opponent. I really do want to help the system that they have come up with, and try and be a part of making it a better process than they have. I just want to make sure that these children are getting what the law requires them to have, nothing less. The school district unfortunately doesn't want me on "their side". I would make them accountable and they don't want anyone telling them where they are flawed. It is sad to me because we could really make a better difference and spend less also in the long run. I don't think they understand how parents are now much more educated and involved in their childrens lives and understand the law better than they do at certain times. The number of kids with disabilities, unfortunately, will just continue to grow.

> It wasn't until her evaluation with the Early Intervention Program when she turned two years old that I finally started to get some answers. She was examined by a child psychologist as part of protocol. The psychologist asked me if Krysten had any "weird" behaviors. "If I had to name just one," I said, "she smells everything." Then when the psychologist asked me if Krysten liked her therapists, I told her, yes, that every time they came out to the waiting room to get her she would be happy to see them. When telling her this, I began flapping my hands, just like Krysten does when she gets excited. The psychologist stopped and looked at me and asked, "does she

flap her hands like that?" I told her yes, and then I knew that was supposed to be a sign of autism, but that everyone had told me she had good eye contact and definitely wasn't autistic. The psychologist went on to inform me that good eye contact doesn't mean that a child isn't autistic. In fact, autistic children can have good eye contact and be affectionate and still have a significant level of autism. After reviewing other behaviors with her that Krysten had, like watching the credits on movies, not talking, hand flapping, making weird sounds, repetitive motions, not being able to tolerate certain textures, etc., the official "autism evaluation" was underway. After sending out forms to all of her therapists and myself, it came back unanimous: Krysten had autism.

Jennifer (mother)

I wanted to share with you one way that my ASD children who developed symptoms overnight after vaccines, have been changed. I tested them for heavy metals poisoning, and they both had it—high aluminum. We discovered that aluminum is a neurotoxin, and that zinc will lower aluminum levels in blood. After only 1 week taking a simple zinc supplement my son was speaking in sentences, looking us in the eye, and able to climb stairs alone. Now after a month, he is still a quiet boy, but you would not guess that he was once close to being diagnosed with autism. My daughter's symptoms also had a quantum improvement with this simple, safe treatment. I have had the chance to share this with many mothers who have found their children had high aluminum as well. My hope is that everyone will test their developmentally delayed infants and young toddlers and those suffering from tics and seizures for aluminum poisoning and add zinc therapy to other early interventions for autism. It changed our lives. Thank you.

Michele (mother)

If you were to elaborate this information to me and ask what it was like being the one with this disorder, it would seem pointless. Why ask a dog what it is like to have fleas or a·fish what it is like to live underwater? My parents had posted the alphabet and the numbers in Sharpie marker when I was three. I absorbed these entities as they were, abstract concepts defining the root of written language. Then, while at preschool I was first taught to add and subtract. I thought to myself, "this is fun!" From that second in time, mathematics became my favorite subject in school, one that has eventually led me to Westminster Academy and currently doing independent study for second-year and multivariable calculus, granting me, a mere junior, that bastion of senior luxuries, the free period. In case you are wondering why this prep school student had a past life in public school, it was because of the special ed teachers and the resources they had to help me conquer my autism. The most significant event in my life was receiving Christ into my heart at age eight.

Vince (16 Year old living with Aspergers)

When Krysten was a year old, she got diagnosed with hydrocephalus and had a shunt put in to drain off excess brain fluid and got placed in the Early Intervention Program for therapies. I asked her speech therapist, who at the time only saw her once a month, if she thought Krysten may be autistic. She told me no, that Krysten had good eye contact and definitely wasn't autistic. Her neurologist told me the same thing. I found out later that that is called an "eyeball diagnosis" where a doctor just glances at a kid for five seconds and is able to know if they are autistic or not. I kind of put the idea of autism on the back burner after that. I mean, if the neurologist told me she's not, then she's not right?

Jennifer (mother)

Jon is extremely smart and loving; however, his behavior kept getting more and more aggressive and out of control. Most doctor's responses were very negative, but as a mother I never took no for an answer. I kept trying. In June of 1995, I took Jon to a dolphin therapy program at Key Largo. It was excellent, I really do not know to this day if the therapy really works, or if it was my faith that made it happen. Jon started saying whole sentences for the first time. His very first sentence was, "I love you mommy." I have to say I cried for days. His behavior got a lot better too. We were so excited for the progress and finally saw some light at the end of the tunnel. Then school started again, and Jon's behavior started to deteriorate immediately.

Maggi (mother)

The first greeting card he actually wrote his own name on...the first time he spontaneously looked at me and gave me the "I love you" sign in sign language...the first time he came up to me and just hugged me...the first time he came up to me and just rubbed my face...These are the kinds of things only the parent of an autistic child can truly, truly appreciate. (I won't even get into the joy of the first "peepee" on the potty.)

Theresa (mother)

SIBLINGS ARE THE BEST THERAPISTS

So do not fear, for I am with you. Do not be dismayed, for I am your God. I will strengthen you and help you. I will uphold you with my righteous right hand.
Isaiah 41:10 (NIV)

I was angry that my brother's mental health was tarnished, and the chance of us having a typical relationship was now impossible. This was something that hurt me so much, and would continue to hurt until I understood the beauty that Zach's life contained and spread to others.

Seth (brother)

I will never forget the look on my daughter, Chelsea's face when I told her that Mommy was going to have a baby. She had bugged me for months that she wanted to have a brother or sister. It had been four years since I had her, that I even *thought* about having another baby. I was not happy when I was pregnant. When I was pregnant with Chelsea it was difficult and uncomfortable. Her birth was a difficult time. She had some early struggles the first few days of her life and had to stay in the ICU, but after that she was fine.

She was getting so excited about it getting close to delivery time of her brother. Chelsea always wanted to look at and feel my belly when the baby was moving, and I would ask her if she thought it was a boy or girl. We decided to not find out what we were having until the day came. It would be a surprise for all of us. Chelsea always thought it would be a boy. She talked about her new brother (or sister) constantly, and was anxious for the arrival.

> Seven years ago, a doctor looked at my toddler son and immediately recognized autism. Since then, I've seen it countless times in the halls of the mall, in grocery stores, and restaurants. I will notice a child who seems a little bit different. Perhaps he's spinning in circles or avoiding eye contact, flapping his hands or repeating phrases from a movie. Right away, I'll sneak a glance at the Mom, recognizing her, even though we've never met. But Miss Manners hasn't come up with a delicate way to ask, "Is your kid autistic, too?" And so we pass each other without a word, just a small nod to show our solidarity. But I want to walk up to that mom and talk to her, because even though she looks nothing like me, somewhere inside we're the same: Mothers who know what it's like to lose a child who's sitting right next to you. I want to ask her if she ever thought she'd shop for diapers for a nine-year-old. To know if she ever sobbed as she scrubbed poop out of the carpet, wondering just how her life turned out this way. If she, too lies awake

> at night wondering what it would be like to hold a conversation with her first-born child. I would ask when she stopped speculating about which college her son would attend. I want to know how she handles the dirty looks and even reprimands from strangers, because her child doesn't behave like the other kids. We could almost speak another language to each other, using jargon like IEP, EEG, ESY, and FAPE. After a while the letters roll off your tongue so easily that you forget the rest of the world has no idea what you mean. But this mom would know. She would know that single word with six letters can change your entire life. I want to tell her that I, too, go years in between dates with my husband, because it's too hard to find a baby sitter. That I've been a mother for nine years, but my family has taken only one vacation. Our time, energy, and money all go elsewhere. Of course, this mom and I are not exactly alike. In fact, besides autism, we might have nothing in common. That's the reality of autism: it can strike in just about any family.
>
> Amy(mother)

She was very helpful and had finished kindergarten right before Charlie was born. She thought he was the best thing ever and would write notes all the time about how she loved him. You always hear the stories about "new babies" coming into the family and then having difficulties with jealousy and such, but Chelsea did very well. She was very helpful and enjoyed watching him in his swing. One of her favorite things was to help me feed him. She would laugh when she saw how messy he would get.

As he got older, they had some interaction but usually Charlie was doing his "own thing" and she would just let him be. He seemed content to just play by himself or watch a video over and over again, pressing rewind back and forth. Chelsea never made any comment about his strange behaviors, or that he wasn't talking. She was just a happy-go- lucky six year old herself, not really paying attention too much to these odd behaviors and such.

When we first learned about Charlie's diagnosis, we did not tell her because *we* were not even sure what it all meant. We decided to tell her in the fall of 2004, a couple months after we first began processing it. When we told her, she didn't really understand what it meant either, but it helped her to understand some of his strange behavior and why he wasn't talking very much. We explained that the doctors told us of his autism and what happens with someone who has autism. Tony and I told her that he has difficulty getting his words out and gets frustrated very easily. We explained that he likes to play by himself and interact very little with others. I told her that we were going to get him some therapy so that he can learn to communicate better with us. She didn't seem to be bothered or worried by what we were explaining to her. Sometimes I would bring her to his therapy appointments so she could see how they work with and help him. She loved to go and enjoyed seeing what he got to do. Once, Chelsea even said that she wants to be a therapist so she can help other people too.

> Having three children in three years was in itself a struggle for my husband and I. Having all three sons diagnosed with autism in three

> years was a completely different struggle. I can tell you stories that may bring tears to your eyes, and stories that those tears would be from laughing so hard. My biggest memory right now has to be when my oldest jumped off the stage at the local talent show and bowed with one knee on the ground. Remarkable because he is the same child that could not even stand a few people gathering around a table to sing happy birthday to him. At one time he was considered severely autistic, they are now wondering if he should have the diagnosis at all.
>
> Estelle (mother)

When we moved to the Orlando area in January 2005, she was so happy. She was going to be able to take a school bus for the first time and wear regular clothes instead of uniforms. She could hardly wait to start. She really helped me with Charlie when Tony had to go to North Carolina when his dad died. One night, I was trying to help Chelsea with her homework and was feeling overwhelmed all of a sudden. Charlie had been having a tough time the last couple days, very agitated and upset. I finally just went to my room and broke down crying. I didn't want them to see me. Chelsea came into the room and asked what was wrong (she was nine at this time). I told her that I was just having a tough time today. I was trying to help Charlie. I want to help him be like other kids and not have to struggle so hard. She said, "Mom, he is fine, there is nothing wrong with him." She really felt that way. She has never considered him "different," she just thinks, *that is my brother, Charlie*. I told her I want him to talk more because he gets so frustrated trying to let us know what he wants or is trying to tell us that he doesn't feel well. She kept telling me that he would be fine.

During that summer of 2005, we decided she would be his best therapist. They both started to connect a little more with each other. Most siblings play (or argue) with each other right away. They didn't have that opportunity because Charlie was not engaged with others very much. He would often stare into space or just play with his cars in a corner staring at the wheels move back and forth. She would always call his name and he would not respond. It was as if he was deaf, but he could hear fine. He was always in his "own little world." He usually always did his own thing and didn't want to be bothered. We decided that we would pay her if she worked with him one hour each day (Monday through Friday). Of course her eyes lit up when she heard the word *money*. I thought it would motivate her. She would also be helping her brother, and it was much cheaper than therapists. She was excited. She made all kinds of activities for him. She read books to him. She would write the alphabet and try and make him copy her. She would let him watch this Pooh video she had that reviewed the alphabet. She made up her own games to help teach him colors, numbers, and letters. I really saw progress almost in the first week. His speech was coming faster, and they enjoyed doing this together as well.

> I am also proud of Charlie. Wow—he has come so far, of course he has a long way to go, but I am so encouraged by the strides that he has made so far. I fully believe that he understands that he is incredibly loved and is a blessing to everyone that he comes in contact with. He is a son that I am so very proud of, athlete or not, I wouldn't

> trade him for the world! God has blessed me so much, but in the respect of autism, it was the spark that lit the fire and made me realize what the little things in life are all about. Had autism not entered our world, I'm afraid that I would not understand how important those little things that most take for granted really are "most important".
>
> Tony (father)

I would sometimes watch her teaching him. She made it fun. She made up pages of letters that she drew, and then next to them it would be blank for him to copy the same letter. She had crayons, stencils, puzzles, and movies. She would do her "lesson" and then at the end she would let him pick a video they would watch together. She would quiz him on his colors and numbers. Chelsea even included a snack at the end of her session. It was so cute and I was so proud. I had worked with Charlie practically everyday and never felt I got as much attention as Chelsea did with him. I was witnessing their sibling bond forming. Even though he had a few words, Chelsea still tried to engage him to bring out those thoughts that he was having. I really feel that when she helped him that summer, it was a big turning point for Charlie, not only academically, but socially as well.

Unfortunately, Chelsea grew tired of their therapy sessions within a few weeks. Soon, it diminished to once per week. Charlie would easily get frustrated the more Chelsea tried to make him do something. She worked so hard, and was so patient with him. We saw so many strides with him that summer.

Chelsea is very protective of Charlie. Once, we had a

neighborhood-community, July 4th get together. There were all kinds of slides, bounce houses, and games. Charlie kept wanting to go in this one particular bounce house. However, another kid only wanted his friends to be in there with him, and no one else. The kid was really mean and said to Charlie, "Stay out of here!" Charlie didn't understand his words but got upset because of the boys tone, and started having a tantrum.

Chelsea put her arm around her brother and told the kid, "Listen he has autism and he doesn't understand what you are saying!" Then she promptly walked away holding onto Charlie and brought him to another bounce house. When we go to Disney World and he gets overwhelmed, she will comfort him. Chelsea will reassure him by telling him, "It is okay." She is very sensitive when he gets upset and tries to help him through his frustrations and fears.

> When he was about to be three years old, finally we got the approval to have him tested through the school board. As expected Jon did not pass any of the tests. After four months of testing the diagnosis came, "Jon is autistic." I was shocked, first I did not know anything about autism and then all the questions. Why me, why my son? Immediately, I began to find out what I could do to not only learn about autism, but how to help my son. I started taking behavior management classes and at the same time took Jon to different therapies. I took him to so many specialists looking for an answer.
>
> Maggi (mother)

Chelsea will sometimes ask about autism and how or why Charlie got it. We explain to her that we don't know and all we can do is help him to be the best that he can be and always be available for him. She told Tony once that when she grows up she is moving to California. He asked, "Why there?" and she said, "I just like it there."

Tony said, "That will be so far away from us and Charlie."

Chelsea said, "Oh no, Charlie will be with me. I am going to take care of Charlie."

Tony's eyes welled up with tears. We have never asked her to do that, she came up with that on her own. Tony then asked, "What will your husband think of that?"

She said, "Whoever I marry will have to like it. They won't have a choice." We laughed and laughed.

I see sadness in her facial expressions when he really struggles. She told me once that it makes her feel sad when she sees him so upset and we don't know what is wrong. Often, I ask her for help. One time, I had to take her to a church youth group event with Charlie in tow. He didn't want to get in the car. Chelsea and I tried everything for almost 30 minutes. He was screaming, flopping on the floor, and he kept saying "No *thank you*!" (That is the phrase he uses when he is scared, wants you to stop talking or is upset). Chelsea tried everything to get him to go outside to the car. Finally the two of us just sat in the hallway hoping he would stop screaming because she was going to be late. We just sat there and said, "Charlie it's okay, you're okay, it's okay, you are okay." Then he finally got up and went straight to the car like nothing had ever happened. Incidentally, sometimes people have no clue what our family has gone through prior to arriving somewhere. We look all content and happy without a care in the world. Meanwhile, we just had a boy screaming as loudly as he could for an hour, while we were trying to calm him and help him. We are often mentally and physically drained just trying to do a simple task with him. Chelsea has helped us through so many of those times. All four of us are a team, helping one another with patience and problem solving.

> I have met only a few autistic children in my life. My opinion is that the more people know about it, the less they have to fear it and the more they can help to treat it. It is a mental condition that effects social development, so society must also be a contributing factor. I remember meeting an autistic man at work, probably in his late twenties. I work at a local Albertsons, and he passed by the manager who I was working with and she teasingly said, "what, you aren't going to say hi?" and he replies, "I'm, I'm not allowed to speak to strangers." She laughs and says, "Since when am I a stranger?" I didn't have to ask to know that he was autistic because he had trouble making eye contact and was fumbling with the groceries in his hands. It took me a second, but I realized that he was talking about me. So I put out my hand and said, "Hello, my name is Brittany, so now we are not strangers." I was really surprised when he shook my hand. He immediately walked away after that and my manager turned to me and told me, "He'll remember your name forever now." I didn't know whether to be happy that I met him or feel bad because I offended him.
>
> Brittany (friend)

I think siblings are the best therapists because they can relate to each other much better than we parents can. They have a connection that no one can break. Charlie often copies her. That is how he has learned some of his language. I think he has taught Chelsea so much already in her short, 12 years. I hope she is more compassionate and sensitive to others. She had to do a project for school to raise money for a community service activity. She chose autism as her project's theme. We were so proud of her. She made a video with her friend Anna, and together they raised over $80 for our church's special-needs ministry. I think Chelsea has taught others about autism, too. She will tell me stories of how one of her friends at school either knows someone with or has a family member with autism. I ask how she learned that and she would say, "Oh I told them my brother has autism and then they told me." She is not embarrassed by it. She is not angry about it. She basically just treats it as if he had an extra toe or something. She'll often say "that is just who he is. That is how God made him, like no big deal." There are lots of days when I need to repeat that to myself. This is just how he is, *it is what it is...no big deal.*

Chelsea had to write some poetry for her sixth-grade school project. The following is one of the poems she wrote.

He is My Brother

Autism is a blessing
It is like the back of my hand
My brother is one of them
His own world inside his head
It is a connection like no other.
I can understand him
Not like anybody I know

But I can feel what he is feeling
He is my gift from God
He not only gives you patience
It gives you strength as well
Sometimes it is hard
But you persevere
You get through it
Although it is sometimes pain
It is worth it because
He is my brother.

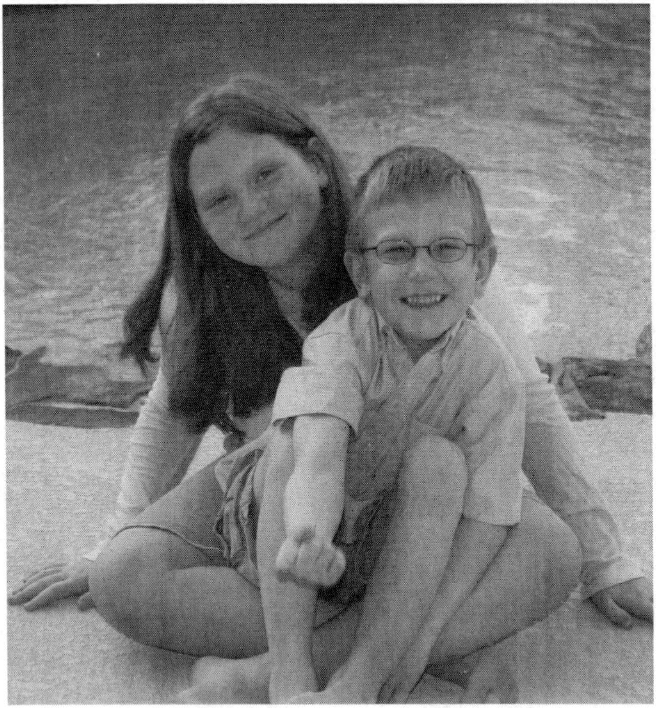

Chelsea and Charlie Dec 2006

When he started solids, he was exceedingly picky about the food he would eat and he spit out his birthday cake when he turned one. He did seem to have excessive trouble regulating his emotions. He absolutely would not fall asleep unless he was held and rocked. He ran high fevers when he was teething and after each vaccination. Then he began lining up his balls and crayons, getting very upset if the order was disrupted. By the time he was 18 months old, he had said a great number of words, but we didn't hear them again. By the time he was two, Matthew mainly cried or growled to communicate, and the happy child we had enjoyed for the first two years seemed to be slipping away. Around this same time I began struggling because I had quit my successful advertising career to be a mom, but life as a stay-at-home mother was not what I had imagined. It was endless, hard work with no breaks. It was isolation. And I couldn't figure out why it was so much harder and more stressful than it seemed to be for my friends who had made the same choice to stay home with their children. I felt unfulfilled and dissatisfied, yet at the same time, I recognized that my role as a mother was the most important and rewarding job of my life. So I started to pray again.

Emily (mother)

It was somewhere around when my child was

six months old when I had thought back to a conversation I had with my mother about 10 years before. We were driving home from the store and she told me, "I read that Sylvester Stallone's son has autism." At age 10, I didn't understand, so I asked her, "what's autism?" I will never forget her exact words. "It's like when a kid is in their own little world," she said. That's all I ever knew about the disorder, and from those 11 words uttered 10 years before, I knew in my gut that Krysten was autistic—I just knew. After all, when she watched TV in her swing, she was in her own little world. I could just feel it.

Jennifer (mother)

My first case was Bobby. My path as a teacher changed forever. Bobby was just three years old. I was overwhelmed but after only a few short days of working with Bobby, I began to realize how much more meaningful and fulfilling my job had become. When I looked into his big, beautiful brown eyes, I knew that there was so much more going on inside of him than he could show us. I wanted so much to connect with him. Working with him made me realize how much I took for granted in my own life. I showered him with praise for all of his accomplishments, even the minutest. I whispered apologies to him, apologies for not being able to help him more. Apologies that he had to suffer such hardship.

Sometimes Bobby would gaze into my eyes and just smile. Although he never spoke a word, I hoped that his gentle gaze was his way of letting me know that he understood. Teaching young children with autism became my passion and I dedicated my life to it.

Tracy (teacher)

He was about a year and a half and the few words he knew were suddenly gone, including the word "Mama." They were replaced by gibberish and sounds that I had never heard any other child his age make. My child was a year and a half old, and he knew every color, shape, including diamond and oval, he could count to 20 in English and Spanish and could spell Monsters Inc, Spider-man, (he called the dash, dash when spelling Spiderman), but he could not tell me what he wanted or say Mama. I decided to go to my pediatrician and ask for help. She told me to go see a neurologist. I was crushed, I could not fathom the idea that my child had a "brain" problem. I felt so alone, I mean no one in my family has any issues, why did it have to happen to my child.

Brandon's mom (mother)

My angel is my granddaughter who is now seven. I have been raising her since birth. Her name is Brooke. My children are 21, a son and daughter who is 24, and it is her baby I am raising, but I wouldn't have it any other way. I knew by the time Brooke was about five or six months old there was just something not right with her, she had starring spells and would flap her arms and sometimes legs very hard and would look up at the ceiling or lights , and I kept addressing this to my pediatrician and he kept saying there was nothing wrong with her. Brooke also has a seizure disorder and after no satisfaction from the pediatrician, I took her to Children's Hospital in Pittsburg Pennsylvania to their child development unit, that is were she was diagnosed with aspergers syndrome.

-Denise (grandmother and mother)

FAMILY AND FRIENDS SUPPORT

A friend loves at all times ...
Proverbs 17:17A (NAS)

I must reflect how much autism has given. It has touched my life in immeasurable ways and I am a better person because of it. Autism has allowed me to meet wonderful people I never would have met, make life long friendships, setting new goals, and appreciating life more than ever before. The elements that have touched me the most in working with young children with autism and their families is the strength and motivation of the parents. I am truly in awe of their drive, compassion, and courage. Each family has, in their own way, expressed how autism thrust them into a new world of devastation and frustration, but also opened many new doors for them. It made them stronger. It made them focused. It made them love deeper than they ever thought possible.

Tracy (teacher)

The support of family and friends is so crucial in going on this journey. I felt so alone at the beginning. No one really knows the pain you are going through both early and throughout. No one knows the *daily* struggles that you go through trying to help your child. No one knows the sleepless or short nights you have with your child trying to help him go or stay asleep. No one understands how you just spent an hour in the grocery store getting all these items but had to leave them there in the grocery cart because he was on overload with his sensory system, and had a huge tantrum in the middle of the aisle. No one understands how you are physically unable to make him leave the bookstore because they have a train set he loves to play with and therefore is screaming as loud as he can, because he doesn't understand we have to leave. No one knows how your other child misses out on things because you have to leave because your child with autism is too disruptive. No one understands how you are scared to call for a sitter, because you are afraid he will give the sitter a tough time. Also, you are afraid to ask the sitter to change his diaper because he is five years old and still not potty trained. The point is, no one really knows what you are going through until you share that with others. They can't help if they don't know what is wrong.

One of the frustrating things for us as a family is that Charlie looks fine. You would not know he has any struggles just by looking at his picture or telling him hello. Once you spend a few minutes with him, you can tell something is not right. He has a great smile and loves to give hugs. When he is comfortable and happy you wouldn't know anything different about him. That is a blessing of course, but also, other people who don't understand what autism is, are sometimes ignorant when they see him acting up, having tantrums, or covering his ears and grunting. We often get lots of stares and strangers walking up to him and asking him if he is okay, like we are abusing him I guess. He doesn't even understand what they are asking when he is having his meltdowns. Tony and I are stressed enough when he does this out in public, but when someone thinks we are not "controlling" him enough or disciplining too harshly, it makes our stress level even higher. If I know we are going somewhere for a long time, I will try and wear something that says autism on it, so hopefully they will put it together and understand why he may be acting this way. I try and take advantage of those moments as "teaching times."

> Autistic people have many great attributes and God-given talents that can help forward whatever element of life they find fascinating, whether it would be music, art, computers, math, science, etc. They are gifted; it is just a matter of finding the gift. They have great concentration characteristics. They have focus and drive when they are "in the zone."
>
> Debbie (mom)

Some friends can help just by being a sounding board. Sometimes we need to actually ask for help in that way. You might approach a friend and explain the difficulties you are having. You could simply ask if they would be there for you just so you can let it out. You may need to explain that you don't want them to try to fix anything. You just need someone who can listen to you vent without being judgmental. Others can help by physically being there, and helping you out so you can get a break.

You need to be specific with your friends and say, "I need _________."

The more you can reach out and ask for help in these ways, the more you are going to help your child.

There is a great verse in the Bible that reads: "Two are better than one because they have a good return for their labor. For if either of them falls, the one will lift up his companion. But woe to the one who falls when there is not another to lift him up." Ecclesiastes 4: 9–10 *(*NAS*)*

We all need friends that we can lean on and trust in such a way that we can tell anything to.

I have had many experiences with friends who have been there for me. Sometimes the hardest times for me, are when Charlie is around other kids his age. When we are at home and he behaves strangely or babbles, we don't think much about it. That is our "normal." Then there are times when he is beside another child his age and I see such drastic differences. I feel there is a bright flashing light on him that says *"autism."* I watch the other children talking in complete sentences. Some of them are only maybe two years old. These are the times that have been tough for me because it reminds me of Charlie's difficulties and frustrations.

> Coopers' troubles started early on and we have been fortunate to have wonderful, amazing people enter our lives to help him and help us as a family. Autism has made me a better parent to all my children in the sense that I have learned to appreciate and celebrate all their successes, especially the smaller ones that may otherwise have gone without notice.
>
> Cori (parent)

The good news is when I start having those thoughts, I remind myself of all the things that Charlie *can* do and all the things that he *has* accomplished that were previously difficult for him. It could always be worse, and as one of my friends tells me, "This too shall pass." It is so true. We could be having a really tough day with him. And then the next morning, he is like sunshine. I have always described it as a roller coaster. The first year or so was like Hulk at Universal Studios. Now our roller coaster rides are more like Woody Woodpecker at UNIversal, still has twists and turns but not as nearly the drops as Hulk. Just remember to reach out to your friends and let them help you.

I think it is really helpful to find a "support" group. There are many different kinds out there, including online or church-based groups. I think finding another mother or father or grandparent that has a child with autism a little older than yours is valuable. They have been there already and have traveled the path you are on. I am currently in a group that meets once a month. It is a group of moms that have special-needs children. I think it is important to me because it is a group of members that gives each other valuable ideas and information. We do not go around the room and tell our sob stories. I think those groups are more in need of counselors. You need to find a group in which you can share what is going on in your life, and ask if anyone has any good suggestions to help you get through those difficulties. We also share good experiences that our children have had with different programs, medical doctors, and activities.

I know our pastor's wife, Gina, has been a blessing in my life. Her son is 15 and has autism. She has been such a great and positive example to me. She has had a tough road but always has a kind and positive approach with autism.

She was really there for me, and listened to me cry when I had those "bad days." I first met Gina when we moved to the Orlando area, and were transitioning our whole family. It was a tough time for all of us. I had many frustrating meetings with the school system and many frustrating moments watching my son struggle to learn. She has given some of the best advice on various issues that would arise with Charlie. I remember when I had started to potty train Charlie in January of 2007. I decided no matter what he was going to be in underwear all day long and I would not go back to pull-ups. It had been about two weeks into this and we had set a timer every 15 minutes to have him sit on the potty. We had our Bible Study this night and Charlie started having his 10th tantrum for the day. I was exhausted and just started hugging Gina and crying. I kept telling her, *I can't do this.* She was so supportive and just encouraged me that night so much. These are the times that we need our friends and family. These are the times where we are weak and tired and need to reach out and help. Gina has been patient with me and very supportive.

> The other day I was writing advice to a mom on how to cope with her autistic child, and as I penned a line about throwing out all the rules you've been taught about how to parent, I also wrote what a great gift that was.
>
> Debbie (mom)

On the other hand, it is great to be able to help other mothers and fathers who have just learned of their child's diagnosis. You know some of the grief they are experiencing and you can help guide them on what steps to take next. In fact, our new neighbors just moved in about a week ago, and we found out their son was just diagnosed with autism less than a month ago. He is three years old. I was able to go over and introduce myself and bring all kinds of information to his mother. That was such a blessing for me. I was actually able to help others, and see how far I have come.

Sometimes family members don't ever really understand what autism is and feel very uncomfortable around it. I remember when my son was first diagnosed and we told our families. The first thing we asked of them was to go to the library and research what it is. We wanted them to be correctly informed. Some people can go into denial and just pretend that everything is okay. I know some of our family always compared Charlie to another child. They would justify his strange behavior and slow learning by saying that he was just like this other child and would be just fine. At the time, I didn't want anyone trying to tell me he was fine. He wasn't fine. That made me feel like they didn't think he had autism, and that didn't help me in my denial either. Most people are trying to help but sometimes make it worse by not acknowledging the existence of it, and trying to make it less than it is. Some family members don't go to functions because they are embarrassed of how their child might behave. I think the more we make people aware of what is going on, and what autism is, the more help we will receive and give. I think awareness is key.

We have been members of our local Autism Society here in Greater Orlando ever since we moved here about three years ago. Our family has been so blessed to be a part of this. Donna Lorman has been the leader of this organization for a while. This group has helped us in so many ways. I have received more information from them, than from anyone else. She coordinates activities for the kids, and it is so nice to be a part of something where everyone understands. If a child has an odd behavior or major meltdown, no one stares. In fact, some people try and help because they are empathetic. We are all in the same club together, and have an unspoken language. Try and find a local autism chapter in your area or maybe you can start one yourself. It is a common place to reach out to others in the same situation you are in.

> I watch as a six year old rubs the back of an autistic student because she sees that he is experiencing stress and knows this technique will calm him. I can go on and on with stories like this. Having students with autism in my class enriches my life and the lives of his or her peers. We don't give kids the credit they deserve for being understanding and passionate people. Educate and empower them with knowledge and skills. It becomes a win-win situation for everyone.
>
> Denise (teacher)

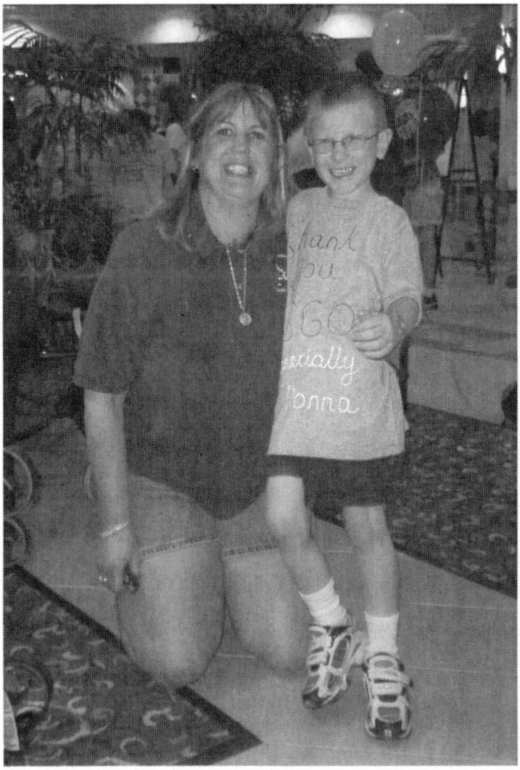

Donna Lorman and Charlie at an autism get-together. March 2006

WHAT IS A BLESSING?

Blessed are the pure in heart, for they shall see God.
Matthew 5:8 (NAS)

Blessed are the eyes which see the things you see.
Luke 10:23B (NAS)

> The greatest blessings are behind the biggest giants in our lives. I believe that, with God's help, those giants WILL fall. Believe it, too, because our kids are so very worth it. Faith, hope, and love. But the greatest of these is LOVE.
>
> Alec's mom (mother)

The definition of blessing in the *Webster's Dictionary* is "the act or words of one who blesses, or a thing conducive to happiness." Within a week or so after Charlie was diagnosed with autism, I was told how "this autism will be such a blessing in your life." I was raw with emotion and deeply depressed, and that is not something I wanted to hear. I was angry, confused, sad, desperate, questioning, scared, and overwhelmed. These felt nothing like a blessing. Everyone in life goes through tough times. After you get through them, there is *always* a blessing that comes from the experience.

I was raised by divorced parents. My siblings and I lived with my mom sometimes and with my dad other times. It was very difficult, and I felt like I was never pleasing either of them. I realized that there is more to this life than all that difficulty that I was experiencing so early. We went to church off and on until I was in junior high school. Then, when I moved in with my dad, we went two times each Sunday and started going to youth groups during the week. I made a commitment in vacation bible school when I was in the sixth grade to take Jesus into my heart and live for him. This was the best decision I have made in my entire life. I got really involved in our youth group and the Evangelism Explosion program, which shows you how to share your faith. I went to Coral Ridge Presbyterian Church in Fort Lauderdale and attended Gangway, their youth activities. That commitment I made really changed my life and made me realize that there is a purpose for our being here, and it gave me the assurance of my salvation and knowing where I was going when I died. I remember memorizing a very important verse which says, "For the wages of sin is death, but the free gift of God is eternal life in Christ Jesus our Lord." Romans 6:23 (NAS)

You can't earn your way into heaven, you just have to repent of your sins and ask Jesus to come into your heart and start living for him. It sounds pretty easy and is easy. You can never live life for yourself. After you repent of your sins, you will lead a life that is pleasing to God. We can't do anything on our own. You can try but it never works.

When you are faced with a diagnosis like autism you can't help but question *why*. Did God allow this to happen, or is he using this situation for *his* good? Someone once told me that God doesn't cause bad things to happen, but he allows them to happen to teach us and to bring us closer to him. I read the Bible further to figure out what God said about "autism." I found a few verses in Isaiah 45:6b-7 (NAS) that say, "I am the Lord, and there is no other, the one forming light and creating darkness, causing well-being and creating calamity; I am the Lord who does all these." So it clearly says that God does cause these circumstances, *but* he will use these for his purpose.

> My little boy just turned four. He has high functioning autism, and that will probably change to asperger's later. He was born at 29 weeks weighing 2 lbs, 11 oz. His existence is a miracle. Yes, there have been all the therapies, doctors' bills, sleepless nights, relocation costs etc. I try to focus on what he might be able to do, and take joy in all the things he can do.
>
> Jill (mother)

Another verse that has come to mean a lot to me is: "So faith comes from hearing and hearing by the word of God." Romans 10:17 (NAS)

This verse was the one my dad used when he did his radio Bible readings. You need to read God's word (the Bible) in order to build your faith. You can't just ask Jesus to come into your heart and live for yourself. You have to draw closer to him daily by reading and studying his word and by worshipping him and having fellowship with him.

A verse that I have taught my daughter to memorize is also in Romans. It is: "That if you confess with your mouth

Jesus as Lord, and believe in your heart that God raised him from the dead, you shall be saved." Romans 10:9 (NAS)

This is the whole understanding of God's teachings in one verse alone. My faith has especially helped me with Charlie's autism. I rely on God instead of things. I have learned that God is in control, not me. The more I try to control the situation, the more God shows me *over and over* again how that will never work. We want everything to go the way *we* want it to instead of what *God* wants for us. Another verse that has been an encouragement to me is: "For God did not give us a spirit of timidity, but a spirit of power, of love and of self-discipline." 2 Timothy 1:7 (NIV) We were created for God's pleasure and *his* purpose, not our own.

I want to tell you how I have learned that autism can be a blessing. It has shown me so much more about myself that I ever even realized. I never thought I was a strong person, but you have to be when you are trying to help someone who can't express to you how he feels and constantly gets frustrated because of this. I have learned that I have patience, which I never seemed to have before. This is still something I have to work on everyday, but I have seen how God has shown me how patient he is with me. Sometimes the process of getting Charlie bathed can take about two hours. It takes 30–45 minutes to get him in the tub and another 30–45 minutes to get him out. He doesn't like the sound of the running water, or when it drains. He has very bad screaming tantrums and flops all over the floor mumbling words I cannot understand. *This* calls for patience, but we make it through.

> I thank God for this boy, for all that I have learned through him. For the miracles he shows

me daily. For the smiles that warm my heart, because I know they came with a price.

Alec's mom (mother)

I have learned to appreciate the little things in life. I find Tony and I counting how many words Charlie can put together. Sometimes we miss what he is expressing because we are so excited about how many words he put together. I will never forget the first time he said, " lay down Mommy." (He was four years old). I don't take language for granted. You don't realize how important it is until you don't have the capacity to use words. I was so excited I started to cry. Children with autism can do the smallest of things, and we are cheering or crying, one or the other. Charlie is teaching us to live in the moment and not to worry about two hours ago or one hour from now. Just live *now*. I am still trying to grasp that.

It is funny that some of the things that I am trying to teach Charlie, I end up using myself. For example, all the time I tell him three phrases especially when he is struggling. I will say, "You can do it," "You are a winner," and "You sure are smart." Sometimes when he is upset and crying in the middle of his tantrum, he will say, "It's okay, it's okay." or "You can do it." I even put these phrases right above his bed so he can see them every night, and I will point to them and say them over and over again. I find myself using "You can do it" when I am having a tough day and it comforts me, too.

When Charlie is lying still in the bed at night or when he wakes up are often my favorite times of the day. I often whisper things like, "Charlie do you understand what I am saying don't you?" Then he will look at me and just smile.

Or I might say, "Jesus loves Charlie," and he will again give me a big smile. I also sometimes just talk to him and tell him that he is okay and Daddy and I are going to help him in whatever way he needs. I always get the same thing. He is looking at me with those big, beautiful, blue eyes. Because it may not seem like he is connecting with us sometimes, these are the moments I cherish. These are the moments I have engraved in my brain, so I can recall them especially in those dark days.

> Having children in general changes your life. However, I have two boys five & seven and my five year old has autism. I have developed much thicker skin, in terms of going out in public and when he has a breakdown and people stare at me like; "why can't you control him?"
>
> Ivana (mother)

Charlie has taught me the meaning of unconditional love. He doesn't carry any grudges. He doesn't think of yesterday or tomorrow. Charlie is always living right now. He doesn't expect anything from Tony or me. I always say, "It is what it is." He loves our family for just being us, nothing more and nothing less. I think all our children teach us this, but it seems we pay more attention when someone with special needs is in our lives. God uses these special-needs situations in life to help others. He is always with us. In Psalm 31:7 NIV it says, "I will be glad and rejoice in your love, for you saw my affliction and knew the anguish of my soul." You are never alone, even though sometimes you may feel like no one understands your hurts, God always does. He is the only one who really knows what you are going through.

He is really the only one that knows everything about you and what you are thinking and feeling. Here is a song by Mark Schultz that has inspired me. This has always been my prayer to my son Charlie.

Here is a little excerpt from his song.

"He's My Son"

Down on my knees again tonight
Hoping this prayer will turn out right
See there is a boy that needs your help
I've done all that I can do myself
His mother is tired, I'm sure you can understand
Tonight as he sleeps she goes and holds his hands
And she tries not to cry as the tears fill her eyes
Chorus
Can you hear me
Am I getting through tonight
Can you see him
Can you make him feel alright
If you can hear me
Let me take his place somehow
See he's not just anyone
He's my son
Sometimes late at night I watch him sleep
I dream of the boy he'd like to be
I try to be strong and see him through
God who he needs right now is you
Let him grow old, live life without this fear
What would I be

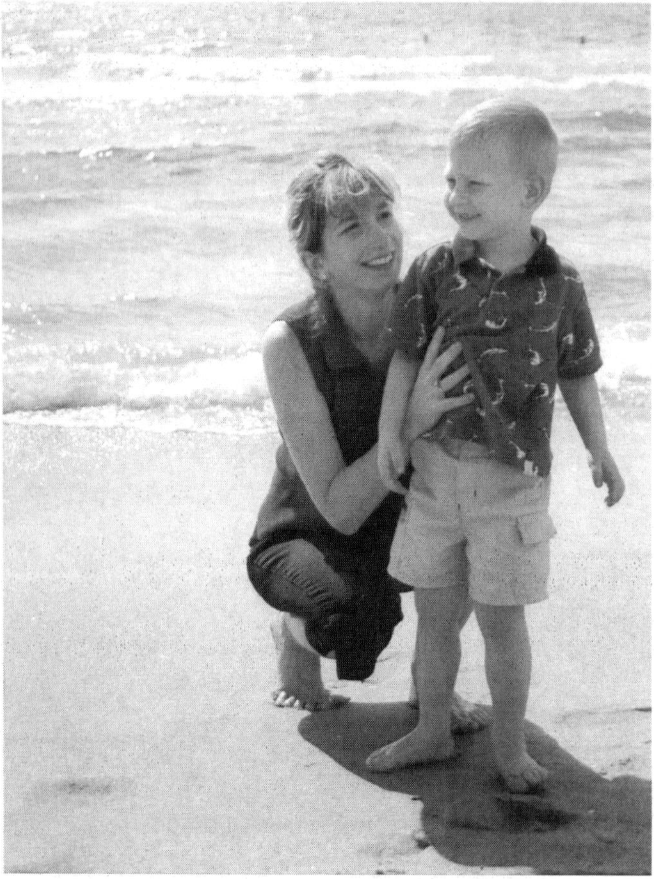

Charlie and Mom on the beach in Ft. Lauderdale July 2004, just days after we were told "your son has autism."

Autism is a blessing in my life because I see us, my family, working together for one goal: to help Charlie. We have to plan ahead on almost everything to make sure he can do it or is comfortable. It has shown me over and over again how God is in control, and I am not. I work on this concept everyday of my life and Charlie has been a great reminder of this.

I love the verse that says, "Therefore do not worry about tomorrow, for tomorrow will worry about itself. Each day has enough trouble of its own." Matthew 6:34 (NIV) That is such a good verse to memorize and say out loud to assure yourself that you just need to deal with *right now*. Don't dwell on tomorrow. We have learned as a family to support each other at different times. One may be strong and the other weak. One of us may be on the edge, and can't help Charlie that day, while the other can handle it. We balance each other out and are supportive of one another. It is a total, team effort to help Charlie, and we are here for the long haul no matter what it takes.

> On April 13, 2002, my husband and I were blessed with a beautiful baby girl, Krysten Elizabeth. She did everything babies are supposed to do as a newborn—eat, cry, and poop. She especially loved her infant swing; that thing was a lifesaver! At about three months old, she started to become extremely engrossed in the TV. She would stare at it for hours, just rocking back and forth in her infant swing. It wasn't like we just allowed her to watch so much TV; it was just that it seemed to be the only time she was really content.
>
> Jennifer (mother)

I hope it has shown our daughter to be more tolerant of others and to open her eyes more and look at the person not the disability. We attend various autism activities out in the community and I have seen how she is more sensitive to their needs. As a family, we use these times to teach her about the disorder and how people with special needs love just like we do. I think at first, some of the kids with autism scared her with some of their stims. These might be odd movements a child may make. For example, some children may flap their hands, some may lick their fingers, some may make odd noises and some may make odd facial movements and different behaviors. As the years go on, she doesn't consider it odd as much anymore. She is a shy girl, but will help in a time of need. She has also used her experience with Charlie to help teach others about autism. Chelsea even chose to create a video explaining what autism is to help teach her fellow fifth graders for a community service project activity. She talks about her brother to her friends and is not embarrassed about him. My daughter is only twelve, but I think she has been so blessed by having Charlie as her brother. He teaches her what *real* love is by loving him.

I think autism can change your family as well. This can be a positive change or a negative change. I heard from someone long ago that if your marriage was rocky before a diagnosis, autism would just make it even rockier. The statistics out there say that the divorce rate among parents of children with autism is more than eighty percent. Tony and I were pretty close before this journey began, so it just brought us closer to each other and to God. Some parents just can't handle all that it will take to care for their child, and the commitment one needs to help their child.

The financial pressure can be tough too. I recall the week after we received the diagnosis. We found a therapy group that could work with Charlie. We had great insurance, but it would not cover anything on the autistic spectrum. The insurance claimed it was a "chronic mental disorder" and would not cover anything under that umbrella. The therapy company gave us a "break" and only charged us $50.00 a half hour. The doctor had prescribed physical, speech and occupational therapy evaluations. He ended up not needing physical therapy as much as the other two. The therapy team decided to give him speech therapy three times a week (30 minute sessions each) and occupational therapy only two times a week. We couldn't afford anymore. Just those sessions amounted to two and a half hours for the whole week and cost us $1000.00 a month. Who has $1000.00 a month just laying around? We did that for almost four months until he was approved to get help through the school system. This is just one example of the financial pressures we faced. He was at the doctor's office or had hospitalizations multiple times for various illnesses like: rashes, diarrhea attacks, respiratory illnesses, and high fevers. Even if you have insurance, it isn't cheap, and it adds up very quickly. Those co-pays and prescriptions are not cheap.

> Jon was a perfectly normal little boy until he was about two and a half years old. I noticed Jon stopped talking, eating the same foods he always liked to eat, did not want to play with other kids, stopped making eye contact and started banging his head against the floor, windows and concrete. I started taking him to his pediatrician and I kept getting the same response, "He is going through the terrible twos." I kept taking him back every month and kept getting the same answer. But I knew better, I was hoping I was wrong, but knew there was something different about Jon.
>
> Maggi (mother)

Some people try all kinds of different approaches. The Internet has a massive amount of "cures." There is celation, hyperbaric treatment, vitamin IV's, lotions, cod-liver oils, Epson-salt baths, and all kinds of other treatments people endure. My only advice on these is to do the research before you try anything. Families are anxious to help their child, but you have to do this systematically. Try one thing at a time. If you try several approaches at once, you may not know which one had a positive effect. Look for the research on the specific treatment before beginning. Make sure they are research based and have been studied significantly.

I know some days I question if I can do this and help him, but I always come to the conclusion that I *can't* help him, only I am able to help him with God's strength.

Only God can help him and I am just the person God chose to put in his life to help him. I have a quote taped to my bathroom mirror so I can read it everyday. There was an article in our Sunday paper about a mother named Donna who had a son with autism. She said, "I never wondered why God gave me this child, but I wondered if I was a good enough mom to give this child what he needed. I had to decide I was going to be."

The first year of Charlie's diagnosis I had such a hard time understanding that I was chosen to be Charlie's mom. I kept feeling so insecure about my ability to really help him. I was going to do it no matter what, but I questioned; did God make a mistake? Am I really the right mom to give him all that he needs? After I read that news article, I also said, " I have to decide that I am going to be okay, with God right beside me cheering me on".

> Shortly after I joined my church, I became aware of special needs ministry and realized the

> Lord was restoring my passion to work with these children. I am thankful for the role the Lord has given me. I truly love these children, and only wish that I could be more involved on a full-time basis. I know, however, that if that is what the Lord plans for me, He will show me the way. For now, I remain His humble servant, ready to serve on whatever capacity He chooses for me.
>
> Denise (Sunday school teacher)

I remember immediately after Charlie was diagnosed how I worried that he would not understand love and would not understand Jesus. I spoke to our pastor at church and he gave me some passages in the Bible to look up, but made the point that you have to repent of your sins and ask Jesus into your heart in order to be saved. Some of these kids with special needs don't understand the concept of sin. The New Testament demonstrates that children are not candidates to be buried with Jesus Christ in baptism for the remission of sins. I believe the words *being buried with Jesus Christ in baptism* means that through the accepting of Jesus as your Lord and being baptized to symbolize that you are accepting him into your heart you will be saved. Jesus has already paid for our sins. Buried with Christ means that we are united and one with Christ. We have been bound together. What this passage says is you have to understand who Jesus is and what sin is in order to accept him into your heart and make the decision to live for him and be baptized. If a child with special needs or a child that doesn't understand that concept, it is told to us in the Bible that those children will be saved. While children do not come into contact with the blood of Jesus Christ, their very nature and innocence affords them safety in the eyes of the Lord. When I really read that the first time, I cried. I felt peace knowing that Charlie will always be in God's hands. In Matthew 19:14 NAS it reads, "But Jesus said, 'Let the children alone, and do not hinder them from coming to Me; for the kingdom of heaven belongs to such as these.'" Also in Romans chapter five it talks about this in more detail.

In the last few months or so, we finally taught Charlie to pray, "Thank you God, amen." He is involved in our church's Eagles Nest Ministry. We attend First Baptist Church of Windermere, Florida. This ministry is designed for parents who normally would miss church because they are not able to leave their kids in the regular Sunday school classes. It has a few teachers/leaders that are trained to deal with special needs kids. Thank you Ms. Denise, Ms. Gina, Ms. Kelly, Ms. Lori, Ms. Karen and Mr. Brian.

From when Charlie was one and a half, until he turned four years old, we put him in Sunday school, but there were always issues. We would always alert the teacher of his autism, but that he would be fine just playing with his cars. We usually got a "deer in the headlights" look. We could see the fear in their eyes. Most of them didn't even know what it meant when I think back on it. Then we would go into the church service but not be able to concentrate between worrying about him and his safety. I even skipped church a couple times right after the diagnosis because I wanted to peek on him and see how he interacted with the other kids. He was always by himself. Once, another child came right up to him and pushed him over so that he could play with the toy Charlie had. Charlie never said a word and didn't even look at the kid. Another time, he was by himself playing with cars on a racetrack and the teacher said, "Okay kids it is snack time, who wants a cookie?" He never even looked up or acted interested. Meanwhile all the other kids were at one table eating a cookie and drinking juice, and my Charlie was still laying his head on his arm on another table moving his car back and forth, over and over again on the race track rug that lay on the table. It broke my heart. His social skills are much better now, and he interacts more so than he did then. Also, noises are not as much of an issue as they had been, and that helps him to behave more appropriately. I think the key is finding people that understand the disorder and can help him when he is having trouble.

If you have a child or relative with autism, consider starting something that you wish were in place, like a support group, mom's group, dad's group or maybe you can start a church group that watches special needs kids in your church. Think of the resources and gifts you have been given and use those. What is God calling you to do? Maybe you have been blessed with plenty of wealth, maybe you are great at sports and could start a local little league for special needs kids, maybe you are a great advocate in the business world and can donate some time to help parents with their children's education plans, maybe you have a business that can donate their time and money to help families with special needs. If you really think long and hard, you will probably figure out one way you can make a difference in the life of a special needs child. You will be surprised at how much it will help you appreciate the little things in life when you volunteer like that. It may also help other parents struggling with where their child can "fit."

> Don't let anyone tell you that the "giant" will win. There is joy in every day if we look for it. Even on the hardest days in these past few years,

> I have found new wisdom in understanding Alec.
>
> Alec's mom(mother)

Autism is a blessing in the sense that it has taught me so much about other people. I had been a person to often jump the gun and make assumptions of others. For example, if I saw a child having a tantrum in a store, I may conclude he was screaming because he wasn't getting his own way. Now that I have had similar experiences with Charlie, I have a different perspective. If I see a child having a difficult time, I now wonder if maybe he has autism. My son has blonde hair, blue eyes, and fair skin. He wears tiny little glasses that frame his face nicely. I have mentioned previously that he looks (at least to me) like there is absolutely nothing different about him. He looks like he has no struggles. He looks like a typical six-year-old child. He looks like a perfect sunshine. That is what is difficult sometimes. I often get the comment, "Charlie doesn't look like anything is wrong with him", or they might say, "You would never guess he has autism." I know people mean well, but it cuts like a knife. I don't want a pity party, but when I hear a comment like those, it hurts because Charlie *does* have autism and we struggle as a family to help him and they don't know all the difficulties we go through each and everyday. It almost makes me feel like they are saying, "Stop complaining, I see nothing wrong with this boy." It can make you feel like a crazy person. People look at him, and there is no outward appearance that anything is wrong. We have been stared at often and have had some rude comments that have been made to us like, "Can't you control your child?"

One time, Charlie just flopped on the floor after getting

off a Disney ride having a tantrum, and some man said, "Get up, Get up!" He was screaming at my son.

Tony turned around and said, "I am sorry sir, but he has autism and doesn't understand you."

The guy said, "uhh, uhh, I am sorry." We need to take those opportunities instead of getting mad and frustrated and use them as teaching moments.

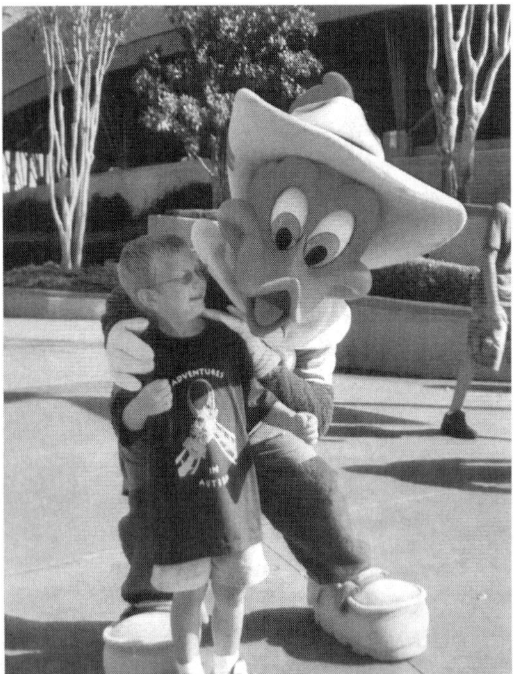

Charlie with Woody at Universal Studios/ Autism Event November 2006

I think the blessing in all of these situations is, hopefully, that we can help other people to understand autism. We now try to wear a t-shirt or hat that has something about autism on it if we are going to be somewhere with Charlie for a lengthy amount of time. This seems to help when others notice his odd behavior. They put two and two together. It also draws conversation from people. Tony has come home many times with a story about someone who stopped him to ask about his shirt or hat.

Tony met a grandma from Wisconsin and parents from North Carolina once while he was wearing his autism clothing. The parents from North Carolina had very recently received their child's diagnosis. The father asked Tony, "Do you just ever sit down and cry?"

Tony said, "Oh yes, lots of times and even just recently."

We have been able to answer questions about autism, and therefore bring about more awareness. Once, a lady came up and asked us, "What is autism?" What an opportunity you have to help another child or another family. We have also been approached and asked different questions because of our autism awareness bumper stickers. The more awareness that we can bring about by either being sensitive to these kids' issues or knowing what signs to look for, the more we can help each other in this journey. It is a true blessing that we have gotten to the point that we can now help others as they receive those words, "Your child has autism."

> To the day I die, I will know this, there was no mistake the day God, or the UNIverse, or whatever power you may believe in, gave these girls to our loving family. Things like this don't happen without a plan. I know I will most likely not be alive to see the final cure of autism, but that does not matter. The only thing that does matter is the children and their families.
>
> Janice from Brooklyn (grandma)

I also feel that autism is a blessing because it gives me the opportunity to meet many extraordinary people that I wouldn't normally meet. I will never forget all of Charlie's first teachers, therapists, and friends. They were the first people to help literally carry me on days that I thought I could not make it. They guided me to the path that I am now on. At first, I had no idea what to do, where to go, or even how to feel. These people gently pushed me in the right direction. Each person, Ms. Sirlon, Ms. Jessica, Ms. Jackie, Gigi, Claudia, Ms. Kim, Ms. Trish and many others, had a direct impact on how I handled myself through this and how I will help my son in this journey. I was even able to meet Temple Grandin when she spoke at a conference here in Orlando. She is an accomplished adult living with autism. She gave us great information and hope. I was also able to meet Dr. Brian Abrams with the Florida Autism Coalition for Education and Services. He spoke about his journey with autism. He is now a medical doctor. He found out his son has autism and at the same time in his 40's found out he had autism too. He was such an inspiration and I was able to hear how he felt when he didn't speak. Those are the stories that are inspiring. We were able to get involved in the Autism Society of Greater Orlando with the President, Donna Lorman. She has been a wealth of information and support. We have learned so much through her example and love. Through the Autism Society we have been able to do all kinds of fun activities that were comfortable for Charlie and our family to do together. Autism is an experience that I can now say I would not trade for the world. It is difficult. It is rocky. It is scary. It is exhausting, but it has shown me way more blessings than hardships. I hope our family can show other families that their tough times can become a blessing.

I know when I first heard the words, "Your child has autism spectrum disorder," I immediately blamed myself. As a mother that is the first thing you think of. I carried this child; what did I do wrong? What bad thing did I eat? Did I not get enough sleep? I spent so many days just reviewing the entire nine months of my pregnancy. I remember wondering if it was the paint that I inhaled when we painted our deck. Was it the Pepto Bismol I took at the beginning when I felt so sick? Was it the tuna fish I had every once in a while? Was it my deep grief when my Uncle T died? Was it the Advil I took before I knew I was pregnant? What did I put in my body that was bad for him, was I being punished for something? These were just some of my early thoughts. I have those thoughts still, once in a while, but I know now that there was nothing I did or didn't do to give Charlie his autism.

I have realized that God created Charlie, not me. I was just the womb that carried him. God says, "Before I formed you in the womb I knew you." Jeremiah 1:5a (NIV)

Who knows what the answer will be of *why* Charlie has autism and *how* he got it? I was really obsessed to know why and how at first, because I wanted to save some other child, save some other parent this tough road we were on. I have decided that I will not focus on the why and how anymore, but I will focus all of my energy to help my son. I remind myself frequently that "it is what it is" and just move on and help him with his difficulties.

> It sounds terrible but it seemed that I had been punished for all the wrongs I had done in the past. I felt guilt that maybe something I did had caused this, and my child would have to suffer for the rest of his life. After I had a good

> cry and got myself strong enough to continue with the day, I called and made an appt, which we waited six months for. After we saw the neurologist, they gave us a report that said he was very advanced but socially disconnected. My pediatrician suggested we put him in an early intervention class. Then we moved to New Jersey. Once we moved I made sure to find a place where he could continue his "therapy." In early January, 2002, he was diagnosed as PDD followed by the dreaded word "a form of autism." "PDD falls under the Autism umbrella …" she said, by this time I was not listening. I kept looking at my son and not believing that he really had a problem.
>
> Brandon's mom (mother)

The biggest blessing in all this is; I have learned to really rely on God and not myself. When you are up against this struggle, everything is out of your control. You are constantly being a teacher, putting out fires, being an advocate, and most of all helping your child. You can't do this all on your own. God has taught me, and is still teaching me, "Don't be afraid, just believe." Mark 5:36b (NIV)

Believe that Jesus is holding your hand, and you can feel his comfort and blessings in the face of autism.

Autism has really made us laugh. My family, we will be out together, and Charlie will do something that will make us smile or laugh. No one else knows why we are laughing. Our family has our own language. I have told so many people that our normal is when we are all together at home. Whatever Charlie does is never that strange or disruptive at home, but when we go out, and especially if he is with children his age, that is when my heart aches sometimes, because I see the gap. Even at those times I have come to accept that this is who Charlie is. Good or bad, this is who he is. That is how God made him. That is our normal. We are okay. *We can do it.*

There is a story in the Bible that talks about the Israelites and when they first saw the Promised Land. Moses sent out his people to go tell them what they saw. They left and saw mountains of grapes. There were so many grapes that two people had to help carry them. They also saw pomegranates and figs, and most importantly they found a land flowing with milk and honey. But, they also saw giants in the land. They were probably fearful. Then in Numbers 13 (NIV) it recalls Caleb trying to encourage the people to go and take the land. God promised he would help them conquer it. The other men were afraid and said, "We can't attack those people, they are stronger than we are!" Then they spread rumors and negative reports about the land among the Israelites. They said, "The land we explored devours those living in it. All the people we saw there are of great size. We saw the Nephilim there (the descendants of Anak come from the Nephilim). We seemed like grasshoppers in our own eyes, and we looked the same to them."

> While Joe is totally nonverbal, he is an excellent communicator. He has an augmentative communication device. At his graduation ceremony last month he actually had a "speaking" part in his graduation, using his device. (not a dry eye in the house!) I have a huge family that has always been a wonderful support system. Until we started doing the NAAR walkathons, I

> never realized how great it really is. The support and encouragement of our family and friends is beyond belief.
>
> Theresa (mother)

They ignored God's promises and relied on their fear of the giants. They all missed the blessings that were behind those huge giants. It is a choice. Do we focus on the autism, or on the beauty of Charlie? Do we focus on the giant or on God's promises for our kids? In Deuteronomy it says, "Then I said to you 'Do not be shocked or fear them. The Lord your God who goes before you will Himself fight on your behalf, just as He did for you in Egypt before your eyes.'" Deuteronomy 1:29–30 (NAS) God is fighting for us. He is right there beside us holding our hands and guiding us.

Here is a poem I put together with the help of my friend, Dodie:

With Autism came a darkness
That brought me to my knees
Then darkness took me by the hand
It said, "Come dance with me."
As we danced I felt such sadness
As we danced I felt such fear
As we danced I felt such anger
As we danced I cried such tears
Suddenly my eyes were blinded
By an incredibly brilliant sight
While dancing in Autism's silence
Darkness led me to God's light
Then God's light took me in HIS arms.

It said, "lct ME lead the way.
I'll show you Autism's gifts.
They're in each moment of every day."
As we danced I saw such joy
As we danced I saw such hope
As we danced I felt the strength
God's light gave me these to carry on.

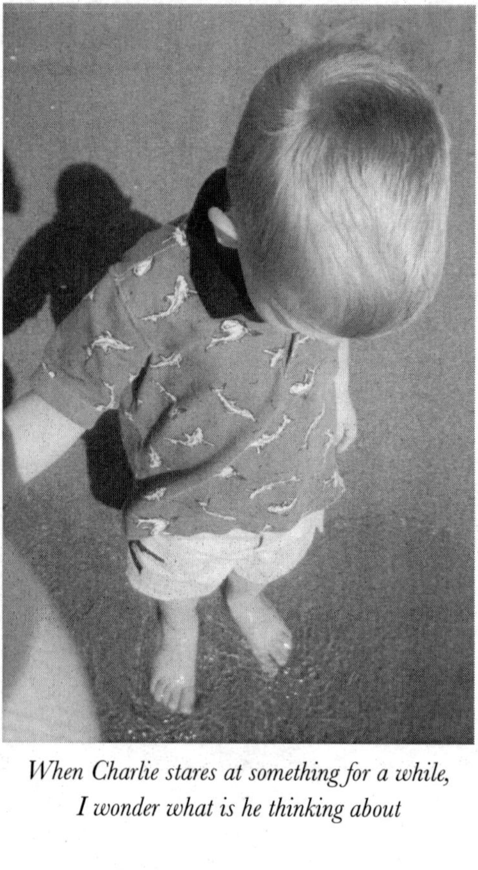

When Charlie stares at something for a while,
I wonder what is he thinking about

It's been five years in August since our first son was diagnosed, and I tell everybody that the blessing is simple...for some reason it was me who was chosen for these three innocent children, it was me who struggled through years of therapy and went through sleepless nights worrying. Me who opened the doors each day to the countless therapists, sometimes having five or six here at a time...but it was also me who cried on the first day of Kindergarten when my 1st son turned around and said, "Mom, you are not supposed to be here, it's my school!" It was me who watched him hit his first home run, and ran around the bases to receive the high fives from his teammates, and it's me who hears the stories about how so and so wants to have hair just like your sons ...

Estelle (mother)

I began providing early intervention services full time, and all of my students were within the autism spectrum. It was only when I became pregnant with twins that I had to take a break from teaching. Even though I was excited about being at home with my own children, I often thought of and missed my students and their families. As a new mother, I could only now begin to comprehend the devastation each family must have faced upon hearing the words, "your child has autism." I am not a parent of a child with autism, but as a teacher and a parent

I am affected by autism each day. I want nothing more than to see autism erased. I hope and pray that no child or family will ever be devastated by its presence again.

Tracy (teacher)

I think everyone that has been touched by autism learns a different lesson. Our lessons were to trust your instincts, accept who these people are, and there is nothing wrong with hopes and dreams.

Heather (mom)

Through my son I have learned what matters, and what is useless window dressing created by society. I have learned that it is okay to simply be who we are, without a single worry about appearances.

Debbie (mom)

There are so many issues involved with autism; curing, preventing, understanding, safety, and finally, quality of life for all these children of God and their wonderful caretakers. I see now how I brought myself and those around me way too much grief. I saw the autism first, not the child. I let the diagnosis define not only my grandchildren but our past, our future, or entire family. Such drama...so much wasted time. Thank you, God for my wonderful family.

Janice from Brooklyn (grandma)

I prayed that God would show me my purpose, and through that purpose, I would be allowed to make a real contribution to the world that would help others. Around this time my mother-in-law, who is a schoolteacher, suggested we contact Early Childhood Intervention. It turned out to be the most important call of our lives. This whole time when he saw the team of specialists no one mentioned the "A word". During that year between the ages of two and three Matthew's symptoms of autism increased in number and severity, and his speech remained substantially non-existent despite the valiant efforts of ECI. He began to actively resist diaper and clothing changes, "squawking" the entire time, and would only wear the softest clothing.

Emily (mother)

RESOURCES

If you suspect any autistic symptoms with your child, you need to see your family doctor or even a pediatric neurologist. My biggest advice is *don't wait*. If there is a problem, the quicker you get therapy for your child, the better the outcome can be. The longer you wait, the harder it will be for your child and you.

If you are given any kind of autism diagnosis, get your child therapy as soon as possible. I feel behavior analysis is crucial. It is the only scientifically proven method to help people with autism. The main focus of behavior analysis is to improve the lives of individuals by improving their behavior. This is the most important thing you can do for your child. Professionals can evaluate your child and give advice on how much therapy he/she will need and they can explain what treatment they will do and why the child needs it. You can look in your local phone book for pediatric-therapy offices. They would provide speech, occupational, and physical therapy. This can get very expensive if you pay privately though. Some insurance will cover outpatient therapy, but most consider autism a chronic diagnosis or mental illness and don't want to pay, because it will be long-term treatment. If your child qualifies for therapy through the school system, by law they must provide it there free of charge. Sometimes, the evaluations by the school system can take up to three months. If that is the case, I would at least get him/her started with outpatient therapy if you can afford it, because every precious moment counts. Also, contact your local Elks Club if you have difficulty paying for private therapy. They have programs to help pay for in home therapy if you qualify. Every little bit helps.

If your child is younger than three years old, he or she is eligible for Early Intervention Assistance. The various disabilities that would qualify are: delayed speech, delayed motor skills, difficulty with eating, or any developmental delay. This federally-funded program is called Part C. Call your local school district to get an appointment for an evaluation.

If your child is more than three years old, he or she is eligible for Early Intervention as well. From the age of three through 21, your child is guaranteed a free and appropriate public education (which is called FAPE) supplied by your local school district. It is important to learn your rights and responsibilities in this process. Make sure to get an appointment for an evaluation.

> Over time, looking beyond his "disability," he was a normal boy, he would come up to you and give you hugs and laugh with you, and accept you as his friend. He never hurt anyone other than himself, he was always helpful and seemed to understand when other people were hurting, even if you weren't crying, he could sense it. I set out to find ways to help him thrive, be it by going to meetings with teachers, talking to doctors, trial and error, I was going to find a way to save my child from being absolute.
>
> Brandon's mom(mother)

Autism has taught us as a family how to be more loving, patient, understanding, and accepting of all people.

Cori (parent)

I have learned to parent my child in the way he needs, without needing affirmation or acceptance from others. Before my son I cared about all those things: making sure I held up the perfect image to the outside world. I no longer worry. That alone is an amazing gift.

Debbie (mom)

It is a blessing from God to be able to raise and care for this wonderful, loving, intelligent child. He has given me and his father so much joy. The best part of him speaking is the first time he said the words Mommy I love you again. Just thinking about that day still brings tears to my eyes. There is so much hope for these children.

Peggy (step-mom)

Last year I was driving our six-mile journey to his autism school, and this child who doesn't talk much says, "Hold hands, Mommy." I didn't care that he was in the back seat. I stretched my hand back there and cried. Maybe he only held it for three or five seconds, but it was a start! While other kids his age want happy meals or dinosaurs, my child loves elevators. We have been riding elevators probably about five days a week for the last two months. We are now trying out all the hotels in the area. He will pick a hotel to try out for the next day. It is his reward for doing a good job in his daily therapies. I am scared, but excited about his future. To me, he is the sweetest most fascinating boy I know.

Jill (mom)

My Madison is four now and little Lynne is two. They are the best things that ever happened to our family. They are charming, fun, and eternally mind occupying. We think of endless ways to challenge them and share Maddie/ Lynne stories together and laugh at what we once thought we would never laugh at. Every word does not cause pain now, I embrace the special traits that make them so enchanting. I learned to talk slower, look directly into their eyes and wait for processing before going on.

Janice from Brooklyn (grandma)

We struggled with the school system. Many doors continue to close in our faces and others remain shut. But slowly, the blessings autism have brought to our lives have been revealed.

To start, autism gave me my purpose back. My choice to take a break from my advertising career has turned out to be a necessity. If I hadn't been at home to tackle autism and all its related obstacles head on, this road wouldn't have been navigable. I know my efforts in raising both my children are essential, and there is not a minute to lose in working towards Matthew's recovery. Facing the challenge of autism together, combating its symptoms day by day, taking on insurance companies and the Texas judicial system, has made our family stronger, and has given me a real sense of accomplishment, knowing that my husband and I are a united force that will do whatever it takes to make sure that, not only our child's needs are met, but the system is improved for the others who follow.

Emily (mother)

Since this all began, I have realized that this was not a punishment given to me for doing wrong, but a gift. It was also a blessing for him because in a way, spending time with disabled children has made him blind to the fact that they are in wheelchairs or that they have trouble speaking or doing tasks. He has become a great example of what all of us as "regular" people should be doing. I find myself being more understanding and patient with people in general because you never know what lies beneath.

Brandon's mom (mother)

Internet Sites

Legal Help:

www.AboutAutismLaw.com

-These are lawyers Sherman, Sherman, & Ziegler from California.

www.wrightslaw.com

-Pete Wright is an attorney and advocate for the IDEA (Individuals with Disabilities Act) law. Go on this web site and register to get his emails. They are a wealth of information about the law and your rights.

www.advocacycenter.org

-This is a great resource, especially if you have ever been denied services by your school district. The center is in Tallahassee, Florida, but they can direct you to the proper channels. Their mission is to advance the dignity, equality, self-determination, and expressed choices of individuals with disabilities. (800) 342–0823

www.COPAA.NET

- This is the Council of Parent Attorneys and Advocates

1321 Pennsylvania Avenue, SE, Washington, DC 20003–3027

Phone: (202) 544–2210

Supports:

www.autismisablessing.org

-This is my personal web site to help bring awareness and support to those affected by autism.

www.eparent.com

- This is an excellent magazine resource. This resource gives several great stories and advice to other parents and relatives. It has some great ideas about treatments and articles that are from other parents.

www.feat.org/FEATnews

- Stands for Families for Early Autism Treatment. This is a great resource for parents. Subscribe to their newsletter. It is free.

www.artistsforautism.com

- This allows children to be creative and use their social skills. This is a website that has examples of kids writings and drawings. The people that have created this site work with all kinds of arts and try and give kids with autism the change to show what kind of talent they have in the arts. This is a site for kids with autism and anyone interested in getting information about getting involved in the arts.

www.walkingwithalec.com

-Mothers journey with her son Alec. It has great blogs.

www.nichcy.org/nichcy@aed.org

-This helps to locate services for disabled children.

www.autismtoilettraining.com

-This gives great ideas to use while potty training.

www.100ideas.org

-This is a web site for Florida residents to share different ideas that they feel need to be addressed. This website challenges all Floridians to become engaged in the policy-making process. It is a great site to listen to others voices about policies and to have some good discussion on what your ideas are.

www.arizonaautismsupport.org

-This is a community in which to share resources and support others who also are affected by autism.

www.prayer@childrenofdestiny.org

-Sign up for these daily emails. They are prayers for parents and for family/friends struggling with autism. Very encouraging and uplifting.

www.autismone.org

-This has a radio program on it with information about autism.

www.autismkey.com

-This is a friend's find. You input your info, and they will match you up with a pen pal. Excellent Internet support.

Information:

www.autismresearchinstitute.com

-Gives different diets, vitamin ideas, and doctors, specifically for children with autism

www.autism-society.org

-They have a "Getting Started" packet you can request that has some great information if you are new to autism

www.asgo.org

-This is my local autism society chapter. It is located in Orlando Florida. They have great activities and information.

www.autismsociety-nc.org/

-This is a great bookstore full of valuable information and tools.

www.cureautismnow.org/

-This is an organization hoping to teach about autism and to find a cure. It is a great resource of information as well. Helps with awareness.

www.futurehorizons-autism.com

-This site has a list of national autism conferences.

www.proedinc.com

-This site has materials that are designed for parents, students, and professionals, and includes helping people who have autism. It is full of great pointers.

www.unlockingautism.com

-Unlocking Autism is a non-profit group trying to increase awareness. They have great merchandise for purchase to increase awareness with this disorder.

www.autismservices.com

-An autism hotline number that helps you communicate about autism with others.

www.autismspeaks.org

-This is a great resource and has a help-wanted section (like a message board) to post questions, advice, and encouragement.

www.unc.edu/depts/teacch

-A treatment approach that helps prepare people with autism to live and work more effectively at home, school, and in their community. Parents are shown how to work with their children to manage behavior problems and improve learning, social skills, and communication.

www.pathfindersforautism.org

-Resource center on everything from medical care to summer camps.

www.firstsigns.org

-Non-profit group that educates parents and physicians about the early warning signs of autism.

www.lovaas.com

-This is a nationwide program that specializes in teaching children with autism.

www.normalfilms.com

-This includes a short film made by a child with autism. It really helps you to understand autism from his perspective.

www.athletesagainstautism.org

-Olie Kolzig, Byron DaFoe, and Scott Mellanby (NHL hockey players) formed this organization to help support, educate, and raise awareness for autism. They are all dads of kids who have autism.

www.bacb.com

-This is the site that has all kinds of information about behavior analysis and what they do. It is the certification board. You can check people's licenses and learn more about behavior analysis.

www.pbskids.org

-This is my son's favorite web site. This is a great web site for kids to learn the basics and it is fun at the same time.

www.fit.edu/

-Florida Institute of Technology website. They offer courses online for applied behavior analysis under Dr. Jose Martinez-Diaz. He is a pioneer in ABA.

www.childnett.tv/

-An internet web channel that is dedicated to autism and other neurological disorders. This is by the Dan Marino Foundation.

www.ed.gov/

-This is the Department of Education website. This is crucial for you to be familiar with the laws that we have to protect our children with special needs.

Books

- *Children With Autism*, Michael D. Powers, PsyD, Woodbine House, 2000.
- *Fighting for Tony*, Mary Callahan, R.N., Simon & Schuster, 1987.
- *Like Sound Through Water*, Karen J. Foli, PhD, Atria Books, 2002.
- *Autism the facts*, Dr. Simon Baron-Cohen and Dr. Patrick Bolton, Oxford University Press, 1993.
- *Activity Schedules for Children with Autism*, Lynn E. McClannahan, PhD & Patricia J. Krantz, PhD, Woodbine House, 1999.
- *An Unexpected Joy*, Mary Sharp, MD, Pinon Press, 2003.
- *The Out-of-Sync Child*, Carol Stock Kranowitz, M.A., Skylight Press, 1998.
- *Through the Glass Wall*, Howard Buten, PhD, Bantam Books, 2004.
- *The Complete IEP Guide*, Lawrence M. Siegel, NOLO, 1998.
- *The Out-of-Sync Child Has Fun*, Carol Stock Kranowitz, M.A., Perigee Books, 2003.
- *The Everything Parent's Guide to Children with Autism*, Adelle Jameson Tilton, Adams Media, 2004.
- *You're Going to Love This Kid!"*, Paula Kluth, Brookes Publishing, 2003.

- *Raising a Sensory Smart Child*, Lindsey Biel, MA, OTR/L, Penguin Books, 2005.
- *Writing Measurable IEP Goals and Objectives*, Barbara D. Bateman and Cynthia M. Herr, Attainment Company, 2003.
- *Overcoming Autism*, Lynn Kern Koegel, PhD, and Claire LaZabnik, Penguin Group, 2004.
- *Facing Autism*, Lynn M. Hamilton, Waterbrook Press, 1973.
- *Thinking in Pictures*, Temple Grandin, Vintage Press, 1995.
- *Beyond the Wall*, Stephen Shore, Autism Asperger Publishing Company, 2003.
- *Making Peace with Autism*, Susan Senator, Trumpeter, 2005.
- *Rules*, Cynthia Lord, Scholastic Press, 2006.

Blessings in Disguise Are Difficult to Recognize

God sends His "little angels"
In many forms and guises,
They come as lovely miracles
That God alone devises
For He does nothing without purpose,
Everything's a perfect plan
To fulfill in bounteous measure
All He ever promised man
For every "little angel"

With a body bent and broken,
Or a little mind retarded
Or little words unspoken,
Is just God's way of trying
To reach and touch a hand
Of all who do not know Him
And cannot understand
That often through an angel
Whose "wings will never fly"
The Lord is pointing out the way
To His eternal sky
Where there will be no handicaps
Of body, soul or mind,
And where all limitations
Will be dropped and left behind
So accept these "little angels"
As gifts from God above
And thank Him for this lesson
In *faith* and *hope* and *love.*

Let brotherly love continue. Be not forgetful to entertain
Strangers; for thereby some have entertained angels unaware.
Hebrews 13:1, 2

by Helen Steiner Rice

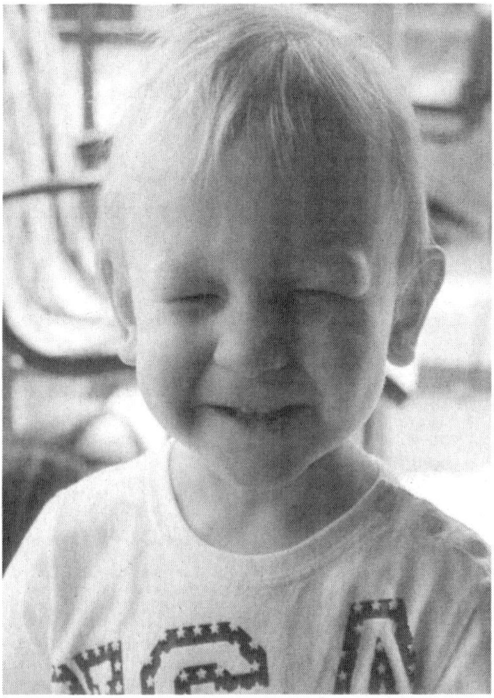

We are all precious in his sight.

The Abbreviations Of Autism

ABA	Applied Behavior Analysis
IEP	Individual Education Plan
FAPE	Free And Appropriate Education
ST	Speech Therapy
OT	Occupational Therapy
PT	Physical Therapy
Echololia	Mimicked speech
PECS	Picture Exchange Communication System

ESY	Extended School Year
PDD	PervasiveDevelopmental Disorder
ASD	Autism Spectrum Disorder
IDEA	Individuals with Disabilities Education Act
AIT	Auditory Integration Therapy
APD	Auditory Processing Disorder
CDC	Centers for Disease Control
DD	Developmental Disorder
TMH	Trainable Mentally Handicapped
PMH	Profound Mentally Handicapped
DX	Diagnosis
ED	Emotionally Disturbed
GFCF	Gluten Free/ Casein Free diet
HFA	High Functioning Autism
IBS	Irritable Bowel Syndrome
LD	Learning Disability
LLD	Languagebased learning disability
MR	Mentally Retarded
NT	Neurologically typical
TS	Tourette Syndrome
PMH	Profound Mentally Handicapped
SLD	Severe Learning Disability
TX	Treatment
BX	Behavior
CARS	Childhood Autism Rating Scale
TEACH	Treatment and Education of Autistic and related Communication-handicapped Children
Self Contained	A special education classroom that has only special needs

	children.
Inclusion Program	Allows the special needs child to interact and learn with the general education population and for the general-education population to interact with the special-needs population.

Be Thankful

Be thankful that you don't already have everything you desire,
If you did, what would there be to look forward to?
Be thankful when you don't know something,
For it gives you the opportunity to learn.
Be thankful for the difficult times,
During those times you grow.
Be thankful for your limitations
Because they give you opportunities for improvement.
Be thankful for each new challenge
Because it will build your strength and character.
Be thankful for your mistakes.
They will teach you valuable lessons.
Be thankful when you're tired and weary,
Because it means you've made a difference.
It is easy to be thankful for the good things.

A rich of rich fulfillment comes to those who are also thankful for the setbacks.
GRATITUDE can turn a negative into a positive.
Find a way to be thankful for your troubles
And they can become your blessings.

Author Unknown

More Blessing Stories ...

What I believe we can do is help them open up a form of communication (and there are many) through which they can tell us what they need to tell us. We were fortunate that I persisted until I knew what was blocking my son's enormous intellect. We've chipped away at that block until he was able to communicate what he needed to communicate to us. He is still learning and the love of learning has been a blessing to him and us. He is not a boy of many words. Alex is in the second grade at a "regular" school in a "regular classroom." Is he "quirky?" Yes and we love it.

Debbie (mom)

Our entire family learned, we endured tantrums, braced ourselves for wild mood swings and went into the bathroom many times so no one would see the pain. But we grew, we forgot about ourselves, and gave all we had to this family that we love. We healed, we were not freaks, just a family who had some unforeseen complications visited upon them. We were interesting, to say the least. My acceptance does not stop me from praying for the cure for this disease. I hesitate to call it a disease because it does not feel like one. I would not trade either of these girls for a child without the problem, not ever! I would like to see my son and daughter-in-law have an easier life but I am not in control here, obviously.

Janice from Brooklyn (grandma)

Asperger's syndrome is like dealing with a very moody wife. There are times when she makes you feel proud of yourself, and there are times when she makes you feel terrible. Dealing with special hardships has not been easy, but I can look forward to the body and memories I will have when I enter the pearly gates. And wish me well with AP exams in May, and college choices, as this "disabled" boy is considering MIT, Stanford, Cal Teh, Harvard, Duke, UF, and UM among his college choices.

Vince (16 year old living with Aspergers)

On the flip side of all this are the lessons learned by the typical children around us. My daughter, nieces, and nephews have learned invaluable lessons about tolerance, patience, and even ignorance. My cousin's son and my own daughter both won essay contests sponsored by NYS PTA about their hero. Of course there are lots of negative stuff, but it is not good to dwell on it. I always think back to how hard it was to send my two year old to school five days a week, but now, years later...all I can think about is how happy I am I did, because of all the accomplishments he has made.

Theresa (mother)

The battle began with the school board. Jon needed one-on-one therapy. Jon's behavior kept getting worse. He hit a window and opened his forehead. A few months later he hit glass again and this time opened half his neck. The surgeon told us after surgery Jon had no serious consequences after the accident and said it was a miracle the glass did not cut any important nerves, arteries or veins on its path. After a little more than a year of meetings and battles we finally got the approval to have Jon attend a private school to be able to obtain the adequate therapy he needed. "Adequate" that is the key word I learned from attorneys. Jon is now almost 17 years old and he is a blessing. We are still struggling with his ups and downs but enjoy every minute with him. He has learned to become a little independent like making his own milk with Nesquik, getting snacks, dressing up, and tying his shoes. He communicates his needs properly, and expresses affection all the time. He loves hugs and kisses. His memory is like a tape recorder. He memorizes every line for every character in the movie. He is amazing, and I thank God every day for giving me the honor to be the mother of one of his angels.

Maggi(mother)

Some parents are devastated by the news, like it comes out of nowhere, but not me; for me it was having an official diagnosis for what I knew to be true all along.

Jennifer (mother)

I must reflect how much autism has given. It has touched my life in immeasurable ways and I am a better person because of it. Autism has allowed me to meet wonderful people I never would have met, make life long friendships, setting new goals, and appreciating life more than ever before. The elements that have touched me the most in working with young children with autism and their families, is the strength and motivation of the parents. I am truly in awe of their drive, compassion, and courage. Each family has, in their own way, expressed how autism thrust them into a new world of devastation and frustration, but also opened many new doors for them. It made them stronger. It made them focused. It made them love deeper than they ever thought possible.

Tracy (teacher)

I no longer get angry or frustrated when I see some parents dealing with their children who are having a melt down in the middle of the store or at any public place. I don't even think about it, I now offer help or a sympathetic smile so that they don't feel overwhelmed by other people standing around. After all, at one point, that was me.

Brandon's mom (mother)

She has bouts where she does not sleep for days at a time, I was so afraid to let her go out into the real world and leave the sheltered life we lived. I waited until she was six to put her in kindergarten, then I agonized over it. We have a new charter public school called Proper McKeesport, and with a lot of understanding and work she made it through kindergarten and did very well, and will be going into first grade. I am very proud of her. She gets speech and occupational therapy at school.

Denise (grandmother and mother)

At first I was at a loss, multiple trips to his pediatrician left us with more questions than answers. He was suspected of having hearing loss. We made trips to specialists hours from home, only to find that he didn't have a problem with his hearing. Finally I was referred to a local program in West Virginia called the Birth to Three program. His "teacher" through this program directed us to a new specialist in Charlottesville, VA. One trip to Kluge and we had answers. Between Birth to Three and Kluge, Kaelob not only began to speak, but he's become a happy child again.

Jessica (mom)

We immediately sought out a special school for Krysten that is strictly for children with autism, and she has definitely made significant progress there. My husband and I have come to accept Krysten for who she is. Sometimes people ask us, "how do you do it?" We say, "what choice do we have?" This isn't a child we found on the street; this is our baby, a child we knew since before she was born. We love her no matter what.

Jennifer (mother)

I am so thankful for having had the chance to work with Bobby and all of the other students I have taught over the years. To my students (and all children with autism)...I wish that life wasn't so challenging for you. You are each so precious and beautiful. Your lives hold so much purpose and I am forever grateful for the privilege to be a small part of it. I hope you understand how much you are truly loved. I hope you know how important you are. You are my heroes. I love you and I am so, so proud of you all.

Tracy (teacher)

She is my miracle and blessing, I thank God for her every day. She has taught me that you can be different and do things differently and still make your way in the world and leave a mark, and this I believe she will do! Sure it's hard to get through everyday, the fits of crying and tantrums, and people outside of our world have no idea what is going on. They think your child is a brat or we have no control over your child, if they only all could spend one day in our lives, they would soon realize what a chore and at the same time a blessing my child is. At the end of the day when I look into those big brown eyes of hers, and she smiles, I realize how lucky I am to have her, and I would not trade her for 10 ordinary children.

Denise (grandmother and mother)

The new obstacles we will be facing will be hard to overcome, but not impossible, now we have to worry about the teenage years. We may not know everything, but we know by our own experience that if you do your best you can turn a horrible, heart wrenching situation into a blessing in disguise. The secret? Patience, acceptance and love.

Brandon's mom(mother)

Garrett has blessed us in many ways. He has taught us all understanding, patience, and most of all tolerance. In a world where there is so much judgment and misunderstanding, Garrett has brought it all into perspective for our entire family.

Wendy (mom)

Kaelob just turned five years old in June. He starts regular Kindergarten at the end of this month. His former Preschool teachers are amazed with what he's been able to accomplish. He knows all his shapes, colors and animals. In fact, he can tell the difference between most animals than other "normal" children his age don't really notice. Kaelob has always been a light in my life, but now that we have the diagnosis and have worked toward overcoming some of the more trying areas he's a brighter light than ever before, I can't wait to see what he accomplishes.

Jessica (mom)

My son Gabriel is four years old and was diagnosed when he was three. I first noticed something was different when he was around 18 months old. He completely stopped using all the words he had learned, and became very isolated. I mentioned this to different people and everyone told me, "I'm sure it's just a phase. He'll grow out of it, just give it time." So we did. Then came the meltdowns, the sensory problems, and the stress! I finally had enough! No more listening to other people. I was going to trust my God-given instincts instead of people who were not with Gabriel every day.

Heather (mom)

I have a four year old stepson which I have been raising since he was just about seven months old. Our little bundle of joy was diagnosed with autism just over a year ago. At the age of two, his speech stopped. The temper tantrums became almost unbearable. We were afraid that he would hurt himself severely. I fought with the pediatrician who told me that I was just an over-anxious and nervous parent. Parents; always trust your instincts. We changed doctors and in the first 3 visits had the diagnosis.

Peggy (step mom)

I have learned to become an advocate for my child, that the doctors and therapists are not always right, and to question them. Also I had to push with my school district to get the education that I need for him. I have learned to celebrate the small steps that he takes, he finally said mommy at three and a half. He now will hold a crayon and makes an attempt to color; he no longer carries his security toy with him, he leaves it in the car.

Ivana (mother)

I think it's healthy to accept the fact that people with autism are who they are and that's okay. While the other kids are running around jumping and playing, my Gabriel is in the corner thumbing through huge books with no pictures. That's how he is! My husband and I will never give up our hopes and dreams for Gabriel. We now know that hopes and dreams don't have one particular shape. They change and grow as we do!

Heather (mom)

Prior to having my son I was not the type of person to speak up on anything. I was very quiet and shy; however, I have grown a thicker skin and now see it that I need to advocate for my son, educating people along the way.

Ivana (mother)

> If there was one true blessing in the midst of all of the challenges and hard times, I would have to say it is all of the incredible people we have met that we are lucky to call our friends. I have never had so many friends in my life. It's amazing how autism throws a lot of parents into the same boat, and because of this we all share the same joy, the same pain, and never once are judged by one another. We are members of a special club, a secret society that outsiders will never fully understand, and that in itself is a wonderful gift.
>
> Jennifer (mother)

My hope as you read these stories of blessings you will think of all the blessings *you* have being in someone's life who has autism. How has it changed your life? How has it made it richer? It is a tough journey, there is no doubt, but with God beside you, it can be a blessing.